HOW TO GET YOUR HEALTH BACK:
& Take Ownership of Your Life!
3rd Edition

Max Stanley Chartrand, Ph.D. (Behavioral Medicine)
DigiCare Behavioral Research
Arizona: Casa Grande

ISBN-13: 978-0-9827756-3-9

Table of Contents

Foreword

Never has there been a more important time for the 3rd edition of *How to get your health back and take ownership of your life.*

Matthew, the man who had only two weeks to live, because his liver was shutting down and he was too ill for a liver transplant, is a good example. Following the lifestyle changes found in this book and undergoing the SIRCLE® program he's been well and back to work for the past five years.

Kristina, left to exist in a wheelchair and depending on her caregiver for all her daily activities had undergone extensive orthopedic surgeries that left her utterly debilitated. After going through the SIRCLE® Program, she can now walk and live independently. Uncountable hundreds, even thousands of such cases are the proof that what Dr. Chartrand advocates here works.

As a practicing registered occupational therapist with a background in both physical and mental health for over forty years, I've not seen such poor health in so many individuals as I now do throughout all age and socioeconomic groups. Larger groups of incoming patients are consistently reporting loss of energy, poor sleep, chronic pain, anxiety, and depression.

More and more people are reporting chronic health problems such as diabetes, acid reflux, irritable bowel syndrome, fibromyalgia, and neck, knee, and back pain. High numbers of patients are looking for answers for post-surgical hip, knee, back pain.

Most of them have spent hours in waiting rooms, and hospital clinics, undergoing multiple and incredibly expensive clinical tests, such as CT scans and MRI's, blood tests, biopsies, only to come out with nothing more than a stack of prescriptions for oxycodone, morphine, NSAIDs, steroids, and other decidedly health -destroying prescriptions. They're no doubt on the road to ruin, as side/interaction/withdrawal effects rule their very existence.

Over twenty-six years ago, I founded the SIRCLE® (Stress Induced of Related Conditions: Lifestyle Education) program in Palmerston North, New Zealand to treat people with debilitating, chronic conditions. These involved severe muscle pain, sleeplessness, neuropathic pain, often accompanied by other chronic disorders like irritable bowel syndrome. An independent study on all the available therapies for these diagnostic groups reported that SIRCLE® stood above all others with a >90% success rate.

Since moving to the United States almost twenty years ago I've had the privilege of greatly furthering my knowledge base and skills through my marriage to Dr. Max Stanley Chartrand, Ph.D. (Behavioral Medicine). He is a dynamic researcher, speaker, and writer who has an unquenchable thirst for truth in research, and I've been fortunate in forming much more than a marriage partnership with him—for the benefit of all.

His work has enhanced and updated the SIRCLE® program tremendously, providing a gateway for millions of people worldwide, most of whom come with debilitating chronic health conditions. Through the "new" and ever evolving SIRCLE® Method they are able to move out of their illnesses toward a future of enjoying maximum potential in health.

Past and present patients gratefully report good news from their primary care physicians as their clinical tests come back with improved cardiograms, A1C scores, blood pressure, oximeter results and x rays and MRI's showing the cartilage in the knees and spine completely rebuilt. Herbert Spencer, philosopher 1820 – 1903 wrote:

"There is a principle which is a bar against all information, which is proof against all argument, and which cannot fail to keep a man in everlasting ignorance – that principle is condemnation before investigation".

I urge all those involved in the health professions to take a close look at this compendium of research information, compressed for ease of reading for all levels of understanding.

Most of all, I recommend this book to consumers who are seeking the answers to their own chronic health or medical situation as an aid to overcoming their poor health and facing a brighter future through an improved lifestyle.

You may have felt that God has closed a door on you...but through the reading and application of the recommendations in this book you may find that He has opened another door which leads you down a much brighter, better pathway!

—Glenys Anne Denyer Chartrand OTR/L; NZOTR; AdDipOT
Registered Occupational Therapist

Preface

Taking Ownership of Your life

How did it happen? How did we go from being one of the healthiest nations in modern times to becoming one of the most chronically sick in less than three decades? More importantly, how do we get back the health of a nation? How do you and your family lead the way? You are about to find out.

This third edition of *How to Get Your Health Back & Take Ownership of Your Life* is much expanded and chock full of hard-to-find, practical, and exciting information. A wide range of research and clinical experience now show that almost *all* chronic diseases can be overcome or at the least significantly mitigated by getting at the root causes and unlocking the healing power of the human body. *Symptomatic* treatment (drugs, unnecessary surgeries, uncountable x-rays) only prolong the problems, and add new challenges. Getting to underlying causes changes everything. *Everything.*

Each Chapter of this new book covers specific aspects of health challenges: why one should *never* microwave their food, even for warming; how one can inspire more adult stem cell growth to overcome a wide range of health conditions; why one should avoid genetically modified (GMO) high fructose corn syrup; the upside on acid reflux and other digestive disorders; the main (and little known) drivers behind arthritis; how to overcome neuropathy of all kinds; conquering diabetes mellitus type two; the truth about acidosis and bone loss; the real health effects of tinnitus and hearing loss; memory loss and shrinking brain; the terrifying truth about opioid pain killers and morphine; benign hyperplasia and prostatitis; what our children need so they can outgrow developmental delays and enjoy a happy and fulfilling future. The list goes on...22 chapters strong! This is information that can potentially change your life for the better!

The reader will find loads of references for further study to deepen their knowledge. However, our purpose here is not to be either exhaustive or comprehensive, but to open the door for greater understanding, an introduction to a far better way. Do osteoporosis medications create osteoblasts that rebuild marrow and make bones and teeth strong, or do they fill the bones with dead cells (osteoclasts), making bones and teeth die faster and more prone to deadly breaks? Our chapter on Bone Loss clearly answers that question. Why is long-term use of acid reflux meds among the most dangerous? How does corrected hearing loss bring lower elevated blood pressure and a healthier heart? How do we reverse the pandemic of diabetes? How do we bring back shrunken brains, reverse dementia, and regain independence without horrifyingly toxic drugs?

Like they say, the proof is in the pudding. Stop microwaving entirely and change your family's diet to at least 50% fresh fruits and vegetables, and see how much healthier and happier they become. There is *so much to learn*, so many things to consider. Every individual is different with different needs. But many commonalities exist. Get healthy and see what's left over. No treatment program for chronic disease is worth *anything* if it does not address getting healthy first: hydration, diet, exercise, sleep, nutrition, and other basic tenets of health. If these are left out, run the other way if your goal is healing!

One cannot simply plaster over underlying causes with opium, prednisone, antidepressants, and heart-stopping NSAIDs. But Americans are literally drenched in them, and wondering why they are chronically sicker, aging faster, and not living longer.

In these pages you are about to discover a whole new world, a pragmatic, doable world, a gentle but powerful world that will help make you the best you that you can possibly be. No stone left unturned.

---Max Stanley Chartrand, Ph.D.

I
Taking Ownership of Your Own Health

"Let thy food be thy medicine, and thy medicine be thy food," proclaimed Hippocrates (460-361 B.C.), father of Western Medicine. He also cautioned health practitioners, *"First, do no harm."*

Thomas Edison (1847-1931) wisely advised, *"The doctor of the future will give no medicine, but will interest his or her patients in the care of the human frame, in a proper diet, and in the cause and prevention of disease."*

True healing, like life, should be gentle and nurturing; not bullying, traumatic, and fraught with unintended consequences. It should address underlying causes first, not fluffing over them by masking symptoms and tricking us into merely "feeling good". Pain is not Public Enemy #1, but is a critically needed immuno-

Diagnostic Cascade Explained

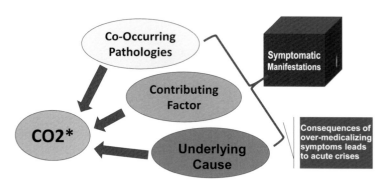

*Note: Blood Oxygen 97% & under means impending health crises.

11

logical guide for one's immune system, Else, how would it know what and where and how much needs repair? Generally, the more pain means more resources sent to the site(s) of lesion and the faster nearby adult stem cells are converted into the needed materials. Pro-inflammatory cytokine messengers make the offended area swell up to isolate it and prepare it for recovery. Anti-inflammatory cytokines pull away the pressure and allow rapid blood flow and fast immunological healing. When it stays in swollen state, it is not healing, but is waiting...waiting...and waiting. For T Cells, T-helper Cells, B Cells, adult stem cells and other cells to rebuild the damaged area—-and a cascade of Macrophage cells to come in and clean up the mess.

Hence, one's immune system is highly intelligent, and infinitesimally thorough. It will not let us rest until one is in top shape. Chronic pain simply means we failed to give our immunology what it needed to get the job done. Putting one's immunology to sleep with steroids, nerve deadeners, anti-histamines, NSAIDs,

Current Treatment Review (US, 2015)

- **Clinical Tests** (many of which contribute to cancer cell growth)
  >90% Idiopathic, Costly $30,000-$70,000 in full battery
- **Opium-based Medication** (addiction, ruins liver, autonomic system)
  Oxycodone, Percocet, Morphine, Vicodin, Tylenol 3
- **Steroids** (long-term: destroy immunology, soften bone, damage DNA)
  Cortisone, Prednisone, Methylprednisolone
- **Non-Steroidal Anti-Inflammatories (NSAIs)**
  Ibuprofin, Aleve (Naproxyn), Meloxicam, Celebrex (Aspirin/Tylenol)
- **Anti-Convulsive/Antidepressant/Antipsychotic**
  Gabapentin, Paxil, Cymbalta, Lyrica, Zyprexa, Amitril, Clonazepam
- **Surgery** (50-80% spinal/joint surgeries leave patient <u>more</u> debilitated)

and deafferentation surgeries does one no favors in the long run. When we become dependent on symptomatically oriented drugs to function, we reduce our quality of life, and dramatically increase the cost of our very existence, and cut short our ultimate lifespan.

For instance, the unbelievable long term dangers from prescribing and taking 2, 3, 4, or 5 heart/hypertensive medications simultaneously only make matters worse. For it inevitably forces pituitary glands to work overtime secreting anti-diuretic hormone (ADH) to fight those prescribed diuretics, by thickening the blood, raising sodium levels, and eventually shutting down the kidneys—that's the shortcut to kidney failure, by the way. Add high caffeine and chronic dehydration to that, and dialysis is in our future, if our heart doesn't give out first. Instead, we should hydrate our body, cut out those substances that are hurting us, improve our diet and food preparation methods, and get plenty of sleep and exercise...and see if our blood pressure does not improve...*dramatically.* These are powerfully effective principles that one wonders aloud why this is not the frontline treatment *before* the really risky stuff is even recommended.

Treating symptoms and ignoring underlying causes may be routine in today's allopathic (officially approved) medicine, but it carries a terrible price: a modern American population that—with only 4% of the world's population—consumes more prescription medication than all the rest of the world combined! To make matters worse, up to 84% of the world's supply of opioid medication (yes, opium) is consumed by Americans—legally and illegally. We are nation of opium junkies, and fail to realize there is a far, far better way. We lose 2-3 times as many people to opioids as we lose on the highways--where's the headlines on that? Heroin use is skyrocketing throughout the United States. Sixty-five million drug addicts in the United States in a population of only 325 million! The highest among advanced nations.

What a sad commentary on the state of American healthcare! Opioid medications should *never* be prescribed for longer than two weeks at a time; yet today we routinely see 20-somethings, 30-somethings, 40-somethings, and 50-somethings with morphine patches, implanted morphine delivery systems, morphine injections, opioid pills, some of the most dangerous substances ever created by man. The reason this author stopped at 50-somethings (on the above list) is that is about as far as lifespan goes when one is on those poisons over the long-haul. A *few* live past 60. a tiny few. It is a virtual death sentence to go that route.

So many good people are addicted that our disability rolls are jam packed with those on "pain medicine". The pain is still there, health is ruined, but once pulled in they cannot live without it. And no, we don't need everyone out there smoking marijuana or anything else, for that matter. The object is to get well—not high. The main underlying causes of *all* chronic conditions are:

- **Chronic dehydration, too much caffeine**
- **Un/under-treated infections (mostly in the jaw and teeth)**
- **Unhealed injuries and degeneration**
- **Microwaved food; over-processed food**

- Too much meat and not enough fresh fruits and vegetables
- Plasticized cooking oils and artificial food additives
- GMO High Fructose, 24-Chromosome GMO Wheat Products
- Long-term Polypharmacy (uncountable die from medications)
- Too much radiology studies (several forms of cancer)
- Too much lead, cadmium, other heavy metals in food, air, and water
- Environmental Toxins in some areas, including airborne radium
- Long-term nutritional deficiencies, too many synthetic nutrients
- DNA/Mitochondrial Damage that can otherwise be corrected
- Psychological stressors, traumatic experiences
- Sedentary lifestyle/Poor sleep

Resolve these and watch children grow and develop into healthy, happy adults; watch workers produce more; watch families thrive; watch addictions and crime and violence plummet; watch seniors live longer, happier, and more productive lives.

pH Balance. Number one on our list of considerations is recognizing that life operates in a very narrow, well-defined chemical range via the Kreb's Cycle. Human cells operate at a peak pH 7.35-7.45. Plants operate on the acid side of the equation—generally 6.6-7.0. The lower our body's cellular pH the more plants (fungi and yeasts) and bacteria (strep, staph, viruses) grow in our body. It is advisable to read the chapter on *Bone Loss* to get a better appreciation of the body's finely tuned ability in keeping our blood and cellular pH where it is supposed to be 24/7. As one can see by the chart below, the lower the body's cellular pH the more chronic (and acute!) disease they encounter. The higher the pH (up to 7.45) the healthier they become. Some conditions, such as diabetes mellitus type 2 (DMII), gout, and other metabolic diseases are primarily pH-based conditions. By focusing on insulin, which causes weight gain (via *hyperinsulinemia*), instead of on pH, and oxygen levels, most people with DMII will never overcome its terrible effects. Little known factoid: true diabetes is related

Cellular pH* vs Chronic Disease Progression

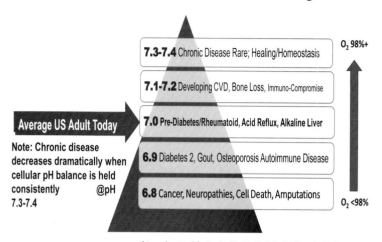

		O_2 98%+
7.3-7.4 Chronic Disease Rare; Healing/Homeostasis		
7.1-7.2 Developing CVD, Bone Loss, Immuno-Compromise		
7.0 Pre-Diabetes/Rheumatoid, Acid Reflux, Alkaline Liver		
6.9 Diabetes 2, Gout, Osteoporosis Autoimmune Disease		
6.8 Cancer, Neuropathies, Cell Death, Amputations		O_2 <98%

Average US Adult Today

Note: Chronic disease decreases dramatically when cellular pH balance is held consistently @pH 7.3-7.4

*Per the Kreb's Cycle (Cell pH & Cell Glycolysis O_2 to CO_2

more to weight loss than weight gain, but because of egregious changes in the American diet and microwaving, we are experiencing both skyrocketing diabetes AND weight gain. Hence, it is entirely arguable that up to 90-95% of DMII could be reversed if pH (and other factors, such as mitochondria repair in the pancreas, etc.) were put front and center in one's treatment plan. The same could be said of most cancers, which typically thrive in acidic bodies that are loaded down with trapped carbon dioxide (CO^2). Raise the pH to 7.4 and oxygen to <98% and we find that tumors shrink—that is, until they are aggressively treated with toxic radiation and chemotherapy—then, if they survive, they can become what we call "smart cancer" and start mimicking healthy cells. <u>Note:</u> See my book *How to Raise Your Body's pH & Overcome Chronic Disease* for a more complete treatment of this topic.

Hyperinsulinemia- Another important term that should permeate good advice on health matters, *hyperinsulinemia* is not only a key component of DMII, but also is arguably the main driver behind America's weight gain (See the chapters on dia-

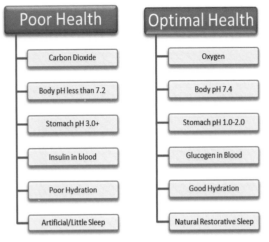

Poor Health	Optimal Health
Carbon Dioxide	Oxygen
Body pH less than 7.2	Body pH 7.4
Stomach pH 3.0+	Stomach pH 1.0-2.0
Insulin in blood	Glucogen in Blood
Poor Hydration	Good Hydration
Artificial/Little Sleep	Natural Restorative Sleep

betes and GMO high fructose). For while insulin is being secreted into the blood stream, one cannot burn their fatty stores no matter how much they exercise! But turn off the insulin, and the body begins to secrete glucagon, which burns fat at an incredible rate! Contrary to popular thought, the quantity of calories is not nearly as important as *quality* of the calories. Once we understand these immutable facts, we can put away the guilt trips, and start shedding all those inflamed, excessively CO2-laden cells that were clearly not meant to be there in the first place! Dr. Barry Sears, in his highly acclaimed *Zone Diet* books, covers this topic with a great deal more depth. Also, further into this publication, the chapter on overcoming DMII will show the integral role that the rarely-discussed *hyperinsulinemia* plays in both of these chronic health conditions. Another, more recently developed diet that is highly recommended in cases of hyperinsulinemia and obesity is *The Fast Metabolism Diet* by Haylie Pomeroy (https://hayliepomroy.com/).

Ions- The "life force", the living part of our food that allows communication within our body's highly intelligent immunology is powered by ions. Until the 1980s, the vast majority of our food supply still had live ions with life-giving genetically programmed activity that made our bodies open its arms to much of the food we ate. Today, this author estimates that less than 15% of our food supply is live. Our children, as a rule, go weeks at a time without eating anything live with ions. Now, I will explain how ions work in the body. The human body is negatively charged. Negative ions (aka anions)

Processed (Dead) vs Natural (Live) Foods
Microwave/Processed Foods vs Fresh/Slow-Cooked Foods

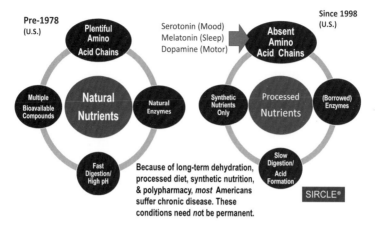

give us strength; positive ions weaken us, but both are needed for the electrical potential of tasks throughout our bodies, just as we require foods with acid and alkaline properties. Calcium with a negative ionic charge, builds bones and teeth through the action of osteoblasts and will not under any circumstances deposit itself on our blood vessels (atherosclerosis) or joints (bursitis), or outside of bones (bone spurs, ossification, kidney stones, cataracts)—all these conditions are the same thing just in different parts of our body. Pace makers are implanted in people who lack enough calcium ions, because today's dairy products are sterile; irradiated vegetables have little life in them. etc.. We did it to the dairy supply in the late 1970s when over-pasteurization (to kill the 1% of lingering bacteria after standard pasteurization) was mandated onto the food industry. There is so much to the ion issue, that suffice it to say, when a storm comes roaring in or a microwaved dinner is served or if one stands beside an electrical transformer or heating pad, the air is charged with *positive ions, making us weak, inflamed, and if it keeps up long enough fosters growth of parasites and abnormal cells.* After the storm has arrived and turned to gentle rain, however, or a nutritious slow-cooked meal is served, or we are surrounded by life-giving plants (which give off lots of negative ions and oxygen), our bodies are stronger, inflammation is reduced, blood oxygen rises, cellular pH is optimal, and we become nourished, energetic, and healthy! These associations, all based on the ionic dimension, are *that* powerful.

Amino Acid Chains- As one can see from the illustration above, when food comes from organic (and not processed) sources and cooked without microwaving, it gives us an abundance of amino acids. These are the *building blocks* of our hormones that determine how well we respond to our environment, how we sleep, and how we are prepared for stress, the things that otherwise make us age. Processed nutrients, polypharmacy, and synthetic vitamins cause inflammatory cytokine responses and are toxins to the body. The chart above shows that when we go the processed food route, we lose the hormones and precursors to **serotonin** (that controls our mood and gets oxygen to the muscles under stress), **melatonin** (that controls our sleep-wake cycle for restorative sleep), and **dopamine** (which provides motor control and acute pain mitigation). Knowing this, we will minimize in our diets that which has been processed as much as possible, and maximize

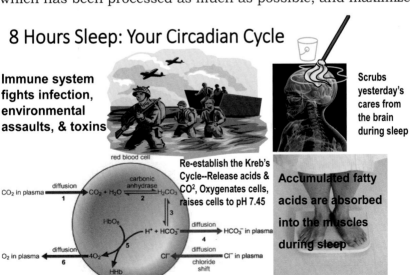

8 Hours Sleep: Your Circadian Cycle

Immune system fights infection, environmental assaults, & toxins

Scrubs yesterday's cares from the brain during sleep

red blood cell

CO_2 in plasma — diffusion 1 → $CO_2 + H_2O$ ⇌ carbonic anhydrase 2 → H_2CO_3

Re-establish the Kreb's Cycle--Release acids & CO^2, Oxygenates cells, raises cells to pH 7.45

HbO_8

3

$H^+ + HCO_3^-$ — diffusion 4 → HCO_3^- in plasma

O_2 in plasma ← diffusion 6 — $4O_2$

5

Cl^- — diffusion → Cl^- in plasma

chloride shift

HHb

Accumulated fatty acids are absorbed into the muscles during sleep

© 2017 MS Chartrand

18

that which is organic and closer to nature. Remember, amino acids are the building blocks of life, and make the food and anything else we put into our body life-giving. Don't microwave your food, not even for warming (see chapter three on this vital topic).

Citric Acid Cycle, Glycolysis Cycle, and Protease Enzymes. These critical terms are lumped together, because they are part of the same process. It is essential that any health publication you read involve this vital aspect of human health. For the citric acid cycle (aka Krebs' cycle) is what makes life self-perpetuating. Yet we have today a food industry, a public healthcare system, and consumer education resources that totally avoid acknowledging that it even exists. When the stomach is of sufficiently low pH (pH 1.2-1.5, no higher 2.0), food clears the stomach within 25 minutes, fats are broken down into smaller pieces and not clump together; proteins are digested via protease enzymes, and the miracle of food-to-nutrition synthesis occurs. Otherwise, we have acid reflux, indigestion, parasites, anemia, and nutrient deficiencies. We eat more and more yet are starving for vital nutrients, making us want to eat even more.

Add cardiovascular, liver and kidney-damaging NSAIDs, and bone-softening, immune-destroying corticosteroids, and we begin to see the sad state of US health. The richest country is chronically the sickest. It is time to get well and get off these medications as fast as you get your health back.

Conclusion
There are only eight categories of underlying causes for all chronic disease. Resolve these and the symptoms of chronic pain, fatigue, lost function, indigestion, sleeplessness, anxiety, depression, and countless other manifestations of ill-health become faint memories in due time.

The following chapters are about changing your life, growing back degenerated discs in your spine, getting taller, stronger, becoming more energetic, thicker and smoother skin, and feeling better than you have for years. Correct the handful of underlying factors and the alphabet soup of chronic disease melts before our very eyes. Diabetes resolves, neuropathies heal, digestive disorders disappear, breathing disorders give way to restored alveolar cells, a slick pleura, and a healing pulmonary system.

Ten Rules of Thumb to Live By

1. Don't microwave your food, not even for warming foods

2. Use extra virgin olive oil, butter, etc.; add fats & protein to diet

3. At least 50% of your diet is fresh fruits & vegetables, avoid carbs

4. Floss twice daily, practice good oral health, fix bad teeth immediately

5. If you are overweight, eliminate >80% of breads from your diet

6. If fasting blood sugar is >90 mg/dL or AIChg >5.6 cut wheat >80%

7. In cases of celiac disease, IBS or gran mal seizures, go totally gluten-free

8. Exercise at least three times weekly for >30 minutes; add BMI exercise

9. Get >7 hours of restful, non-medicated sleep nightly, take short nap daily

10. Make water your main source of hydration, go moderate on caffeine

DigiCare® Behavioral Research, 2015

Use Deep Cold Laser instead of surgery for most lesions and degeneration; stimulate adult stem cells instead of taking more medication; overcome nutrient deficiencies with the food we eat instead of a handful of toxic, synthetic substitutes. Drink purified, alkalized, ionized water instead of adding poisonous chemicals like chlorine and fluorides. Avoid plasticized cooking oils like Canola Oil and go for Omega-9 rich Extra Virgin Olive Oil. Avoid GMO wheat like the plague; and refuse to eat or drink foods with GMO High Fructose Corn Syrup and we will not suffer as many of the avoidable ailments we see all around us.

Instead, we will enjoy long life and the highest quality of life possible. It's called taking charge of our life, not leaving it to those who would merely "manage" our health.

II
TRUE HEALING:

The Future is Now For Those Who Truly Want It

Deep Cold Laser, Medical Massage, Nutrition, Essential Oils, SOQI
Wellness Technology, Video Otoscopy, Occupational & Much More!

Introduction: *This book is about true healing that involves a specially trained and coordinated team, even a Community Healthcare Team, using the latest gentle yet powerful modalities that. The team includes everything listed above in the subtitle, plus: conservative integrative medicine physicians, oral surgeons, dentists, nutritionists, physical therapists, chiropractors, acupuncturists, mental health counselors, audiologists, hearing aid specialists, deaf educators, speech pathologists, research-practitioners, nurses, pulmonologists, and more. In addition to deep cold laser (which is fast replacing the need for many surgeries), medical massage, SOQI Wellness Technology, video otoscopy, and occupational therapy, you'll find inversion tables, negative ion generators, BMI exercise (vibration plate), ionized/alkalized water, etc. Opioids and the really bad stuff are reserved for traumas and acute episodes; certainly not for long-term chronic problems. Throughout this book, you are about to discover how all diagnostic and prescriptive roads should lead back to healing. To be sure, just about all disease known to man can be overcome, lessened, and managed—drats, there we said it: "managed". "Management of disease" is the mainstay of today's medicine. It should instead be the rare last resort, the road less traveled, the way it works only until we find a way to resolve the problem, once and for all! As a healing profession, we should never stop at managing, period. Healing should ever be the goal.*

Introducing Deep Cold Laser

Advanced Therapeutic III-b Deep Cold Laser is an FDA-approved modality that heals, not just manages, a wide variety of conditions. It has a solid record of safety in the hands of a trained Certified Cold Laser Therapist and Occupational Therapist. *Deep Cold Laser or even standard laser should never be used by consumers. The risks of serious and severe mitochondrial harm are just too great. As the technology improves, and the effects become more powerful, this caution becomes more imperative.*

Deep Cold Laser differs from standard laser in several ways, the most apparent of which is that it utilizes controlled monochromatic light at the frequency of 830 nanometers (nm) as the optimal therapeutic window. In this region the captured light penetrates more deeply into the tissues of the body, stimulating mitochondria of the targeted region. More and more, 830 nm low

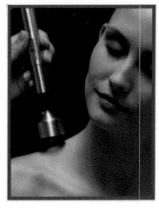

level laser light is often supplemented with other red and infra-red, even far infrared, frequencies and with improved therapeutic strategies to speed or concentrate photons. Pulsed forms are safer but not as aggressive. Non-pulsed forms are more aggressive but require special care in how it is administered, especially if the objective is in resolving bone spurs, frozen joints, and heterotopic ossification as often happens post-surgically and from traumatic and unhealed injuries, or from long-term subclinical exposure to sepsis, such as from teeth and jaw, or from parasitic wastes along the spine or lower legs in the interstitial spaces.

The stimulating effect of photons on enzymes and Adenosine Triphosphate (ATP) in the mitochondria causes secretion of

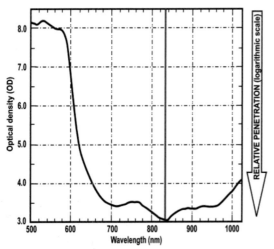

serotonin as the marker neurotransmitter for as long as there is adequate oxygen for the mitochondria to convert into adenosine triphosphate (ATP) that is transferred into healing energy.

This, in turn, causes an "enzyme

cascade" that excites light-sensitive cyto-chromes, provides nearby adult stem cells the extra energy need-ed to grow, regenerate, and to heal at an in-credibly faster rate than by any other clinical method. Be-sides focused stimu-lation at a given site, the most important goal is getting mas-sive amounts of blood to the site of lesion, along with the needed T-cells, T Helper-cells, B-cells, and large, lumbering macro-phage cells to clean up the mess and make way for hemo-globin and red cells to bring life-empowering oxygen to the site. So powerful is this pro-cess that it requires

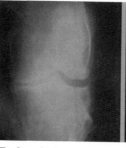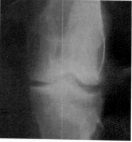

Before/After Knee Cartilage Regeneration @ 12 weeks. Similar results in cases of degenerated spinal discs.

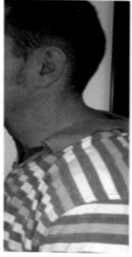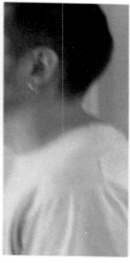

Before & After: Auto accident victim resolved headaches, neuropathy, spinal stenosis, severe tachycardia, and regained 2" in height.

up to 90% of the energy you get from the food you digest while you are under treatment! Nothing heals faster than appropri-ately administered cold laser when utilized with nutritional building blocks obtained only from organic and readily usable sources. Medications generally slow down this process and prolong the time it takes to heal.

Deep Cold laser, used as a stand alone therapy does little more than reduce inflammation at the site. But when used in

23

a program like the trademarked SIRCLE® Program Deep Cold Laser that utilizes several powerful adjunctive therapies and building blocks to properly prepare the site of lesion, one can be assured of enjoying the most stimulating, longest lasting Deep Cold Laser in use today. This is one reason that results vary so much in widely disparate studies on cold laser. Despite differences in levels of preparation and application, few healing technologies have been studied as thoroughly as cold laser technology. While cold laser has been around since around 1954, it was not until the mid-2000s onward that the public has been able to start enjoying the benefits of cold laser in widespread clinical settings.

When the cold laser described here is used in its most complete context—patient stops microwaving food, reduces medications as much as is safe and under professional guidance, overcomes dehydration and all possible nutrition deficiencies, resolves all subclinical infections (especially tooth and jaw sepsis), exercises and gets plenty of restful sleep (not drugged sleep), AND enjoys adjunctive therapies prior to lasering—such as medical massage, SOQI, and essential oils—every single DCL treatment program is a winner in its own right. Results are incredible compared to any other modality in use today. It then becomes, by definition, *Deep* Cold Laser.

Using Deep Cold Laser, used in this way, reduces the need for debilitating non-steroidal anti-inflammatory drugs (NSAIDs), such as Naproxyn, Ibuprofen, etc., or dangerously addictive opioid pain killers, such as Oxycodone, Oxycontin, Morphine, Tylenol 3, Percocet, Dilaudid, etc., for more rapid recovery from a wide variety of injuries & conditions:

- *Muscle strains/sprains*, *ligament/tendon injuries, open wounds/bone injuries, fractures, joint dysfunction & bone spurs (osteophytes).*
- *Neural conditions*, *such as diabetic, peripheral & idiopathic neuropathies, fibromyalgia, multiple sclerosis, neuralgia, and restless leg syndrome.*
- *Neck & back pain*, *for faster, more permanent relief within a specially designed rehabilitation program.*
- *Knee, leg and feet pain*, *along with a recommended nutritional supplement program that restores function while it re-*

SIRCLE® Medical Massage & Aroma- Touch® Therapies with Deep Cold Laser

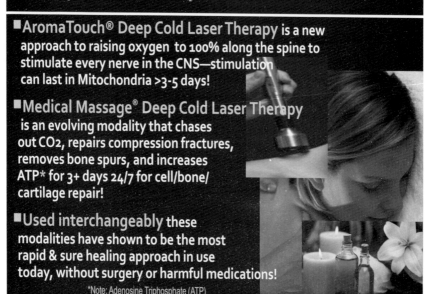

- ■AromaTouch® Deep Cold Laser Therapy is a new approach to raising oxygen to 100% along the spine to stimulate every nerve in the CNS—stimulation can last in Mitochondria >3-5 days!

- ■Medical Massage® Deep Cold Laser Therapy is an evolving modality that chases out CO_2, repairs compression fractures, removes bone spurs, and increases ATP* for 3+ days 24/7 for cell/bone/cartilage repair!

- ■Used interchangeably these modalities have shown to be the most rapid & sure healing approach in use today, without surgery or harmful medications!

*Note: Adenosine Triphosphate (ATP)

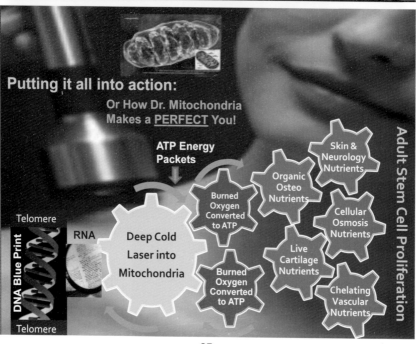

Putting it all into action:

Or How Dr. Mitochondria Makes a **PERFECT** You!

ATP Energy Packets

Deep Cold Laser into Mitochondria

Burned Oxygen Converted to ATP

Burned Oxygen Converted to ATP

Organic Osteo Nutrients

Skin & Neurology Nutrients

Cellular Osmosis Nutrients

Live Cartilage Nutrients

Chelating Vascular Nutrients

Telomere

RNA

DNA Blue Print

Telomere

Adult Stem Cell Proliferation

lieves pain.

- **Failed surgeries**, or in cases of recovery-delaying cortisone injections.

Deep Cold Laser is best used for localized pain, i.e.: of the Neck, Shoulder, Back, Knees, Feet, Hands, or in cases of: Fibromyalgia, Rheumatoid Arthritis, Multiple Sclerosis/ALS, Repetitive Strain Injuries, Carpal Tunnel Syndrome, Ankylosing Spondylitis, Pinched Nerves, Herniated or Bulging Discs, Neuropathies, Migraine Headaches, Digestive Disorders, Breathing Disorders, and Much, Much More!

Introducing Deep *Truly Effective* Cold Laser

Deep Cold Laser Goes Deep & Lasts Long...*if:*

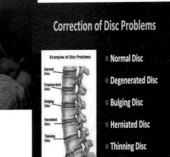

Correction of Disc Problems

Examples of Disc Problems
- Normal Disc
- Degenerated Disc
- Bulging Disc
- Herniated Disc
- Thinning Disc
- Osteophyte (Spurs)

- There's enough O_2 at site of lesion
- CO_2, Toxins are first removed
- Cellular pH is @ 7.3-7.45, O_2 <98%
- Taking organic building blocks for repair of cartilage, bone, soft tissues, vascularization
- Resolution of subclinical infections. Including tooth/jaw sepsis
- Resolution of unhealed injuries, stenosis, compression fractures

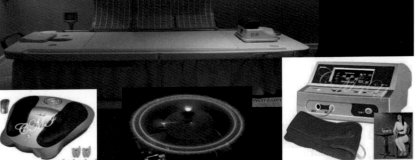

The SOQI Wellness Lab®:
Gentle & Powerfully Healing

26

Gateway to your journey: A Free Video Otoscopy Biomarker Assessment*

Assess your health history relative to:

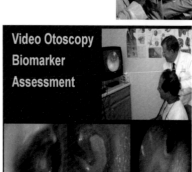

- ☐ Bone & joint integrity
- ☐ Cartilage integrity:
    clear hyaline, soft white, fibrocartilage
- ☐ Cardiovascular status:
    micro & macro systems
- ☐ Epithelial, Neurological health
- ☐ Hydration & cellular pH
- ☐ Neurological Status

☐

*Research-based approach for a complete health assessment developed over a period of 40+ years by Dr. Chartrand & Associates

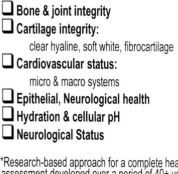

What health professionals have said about the seminars and in-service training given by Dr. Chartrand on these topics

-*"I practiced medicine for almost 40 years before retiring, and now wish I knew during that time what I learned from you at last night's seminar !"*

"As a nurse practitioner I've found a wealth of knowledge we are just not being taught in nursing school. I feel I can be of so much more help to my patients now that I see the larger picture from your seminars!"

"I knew periodontal health was important. But I never imagined that conditions like rheumatoid arthritis and depression were caused more from sepsis trapped in teeth and jaws than any other cause. You've given me a much greater appreciation for the lifesaving work I do with my dental patients!"

"You've shown me how many of my chiropractic patients need their treatment program supplemented with what you do at SIRCLE. Without these, the relief I give them may only be temporary."

Note to Reader: Relative to statements made here about the above mentioned modalities, the FDA has evaluated and approved some of the statements, such as those pertaining to the 830 nm cold laser, while other aspects of application may not have been evaluated. Essential oils referred to here are generally regarded as safe (GRAS) when used appropriately. SOQI Wellness technologies are considered FDA Class I medical devices and have been evaluated and accepted in certain other nations as Class II devices. The benefits of medical massage are well documented in the literature. However, the descriptions used in this book pertaining to these and other technologies do not constitute a diagnosis or treatment in individual cases. It is always advisable to consult with licensed health professionals in matters of health and prescription medications.

III

Understanding Adult Stem Cells
The Very Key for Repair of Injuries, Degeneration, Infections & Toxins

Introduction: The more we learn about Adult Stem Cells (ASCs) and what they do, the more we realize that they are the very key to repairing and rejuvenating the human body from old injuries, past infections, and long-term toxic exposure. Indeed, as *telomeres* are strengthened, *Deoxyribonucleic Acid (DNA)* strands lengthened, and the energy of *Adenosine Triphosphate (ATP)* is brought to a roaring blaze by laser-stimulated *Mitochondria*, ASCs slow (and reverse) the aging process, and restore us closer to the ideal of our DNA blueprint. Treatments, supplementation, and lifestyle changes that bring out and direct more ASCs in a given patient should be the objective of every worthwhile clinical approach. Hence, a wide array of therapies and practices could fit into the ASC template. Our purpose here is to present a brief review of the natural systems that are set in motion when we take advantage of the body's own ability to restore our body's health and well-being.

DNA: Your Genome "Time Capsule"

In 1886, biologist Robert Altmann saw for the first time under a microscope what he called "bioblasts" or "the engines of life". These "engines" were organelles called **Mitochondria** and the energy they generated is called **adenosine triphosphate (ATP)**.

It was not until the invention of electron microscopy in 1962 that scientists were able to actually see the microscopic components of these "little animals" (as they were called by earlier scientists from the nineteenth century). Mitochondria, they

29

discovered, are microscopic organelles of *foreign* origin that contain their own DNA apart from our body's own DNA. In fact, they are the only organelle in the human body that is *not* an original part of us. We cannot live without them for more than mere minutes, yet they can turn on us on a dime and wreak the havoc we call *autoimmune disease* when conditions are less than to their liking (low cellular pH, environmental toxins, or deficiency in oxygen, water, and nutrients).

The mission of Mitochondria is to read our DNA Blueprint and keep our cells matching the specifications of the blue print. When we are children it assures that we develop to our fullest potential; when we are older it reaches back in time and strives to maintain us to our original DNA specifications.

One's DNA record represents what I call our **"Human Genome Time Capsule"**, meaning our genes are the product of the survivors of our bloodline—the "best of the best", if you will. We were not destined to be sickly, spend our last ten years of life in convalescence or on umpteen side effect laden medications. We were meant to maintain robust health by empowering the body's far superior immunological and restorative processes to the very end of life itself. Indeed we were

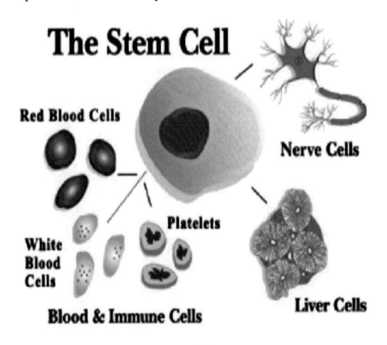

The Stem Cell

Red Blood Cells

Nerve Cells

Platelets

White Blood Cells

Blood & Immune Cells

Liver Cells

The SIRCLE® Method is based on *how* the body regenerates tissues for maintenance & repair

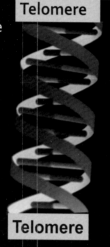

Telomere

- **Mitochondria:** The "doctor" in every cell-burns >90% of the energy from the food you eat to make ATP, the crew that carries out repair/regeneration under the direction of mitochondria

- **RNA:** DNA translator for Dr. Mitochondria

- **DNA Blueprint:** A genetic map of a perfect you!

- **Telomeres:** The "shoelace ends of the DNA"

- **Stem Cells:** Building blocks for regeneration

*Current Research: Strengthening telomeres can add as much as 10-15 years to one's lifespan

Telomere

meant to pass on to the next generation an enhanced and improved genetic roadmap for them to follow.

Enter Adult Stem Cells

So, the Mitochondria of our cells produce "energy packets" called ATP, which search for the missing elements required to make us whole. Our immunology guides the ATP by alerting where bone, cartilage, soft tissues, etc. need repair—often detected in the form of pain and/or inflammation.

ATP relies upon messengers called **Cytokines** to guide its work. If we're healing, anti-inflammatory cytokines will be released. If we're *not*, proinflammatory cytokines will be released. When the proinflammatory kind are released, an entire cascade of restorative processes are set in motion. But if we artificially turn off proinflammatory cytokines with, say, long term prednisone or addictive opioid pain medication, the healing process stops and we continue to decline while being none the wiser of our true health state.

To empower the Adult Stem Cells (ASCs) to convert into the needed tissue (cartilage, bone, myelin, skin, blood vessels, etc.) one must have supplementation of the building blocks or nutrients to finish the ASC conversion process. Once that happens, and attention to the site of lesion is fostered by deep cold laser, medical massage, medical grade essential oils, negative ion pulses, and other gentle therapies, healing begins and will continue 24/7 until 1) the therapeutic stimulus ceases, or 2) the Mitochondria receive immunological signals that the injured site now matches the DNA blueprint.

An example of this is: no matter how damaging the injury one might incur on their fingers, short of amputation or severe burn, their fingerprint will always grow back according to one's DNA blueprint! In the case of degenerated discs of the spine, worn cartilage in the knees, destruction of bone in the hips or shoulders, or even serious neuropathy of the legs and feet, the good news is that under an effective treatment program, one's ASCs can repair just about any and all of the damage and return the body back to a fully functioning state better than surgery or drugs could begin to accomplish.

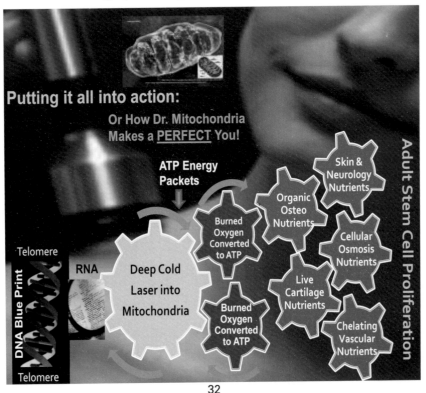

Note: Monographs by Dr. Chartrand cover hundreds of topics explaining how one may benefit from adult stem cell healing with cutting edge treatment approaches. For more information, contact: DigiCare Behavioral Research, 820 W. Cottonwood Lane, Suite #6, Casa Grande, AZ 85122, (520)509-6380.

Resources for Further Study

Chakkalakal, JV, Jones, KM, Basson, MA, Brack, AS (2012). The Aged Niche Disrupts Stem Muscle Cell Quiescence. *Nature, 490*, 355-360.

Chartrand, MS (2013). *Dr. Mitochondria & You* (DVD Seminar Lecture). Casa Grande, AZ: DigiCare.

Chartrand, MS (2015). *Understanding how your own adult stem cells provide healing from injury and degeneration*, (DVD Version) Casa Grande, AZ: DigiCare.

Felcon, W. (2006). Stem Cell Therapy in a Pill? *Life Extension, December*, http://stemcells.nih.gov/staticresources/info/basics/StemCellBasics.pdf

Gnecchi, M., Zhang, Z., Ni, A, and Dzau, V (2008). Paracrine mechanisms in Adult Stem Cell Signaling and Therapy. *Circulation Research*, http://circres.ahajournals.org/content/103/11/1204.full

Jensen, FE, et al. (1994). The putative essential nutrient pyrroloquinoline quinone is a neuroprotective in a rodent model of hypoxic/ischemic brain injury. Neuroscience, 62: 2 or http://www.sciencedirect.com/science/article/pii/0306452294903751

National Institutes of Health (2014). Stem Cell Information. http://stemcells.nih.gov/staticresources/info/basics/StemCellBasics.pdf

Yu, Q., Y.S. Bai, and J. Lin, (2010). Effect of astragalus injection combined with mesenchymal stem cells transplantation for repairing the Spinal cord injury in rats. *Zhongguo Zhong Xi Yi Jie He Za Zhi*, 30(4): p. 393-7.

IV
But what's wrong with
MICROWAVING?

Introduction: *Public health researchers have tried mightily to explain why every category of chronic disease in the US is at pandemic proportions and getting worse by the day. Diabetes Type II (DMII), cardiovascular disease (CVD), Cancer, Neuropathies, and now Alzheimer's disease (AD). These have all grown manifold per capita since 1970 and each disease has spawned huge investor-owned industries worth trillions of dollars that*

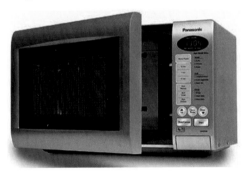

would collapse if people were to change their diet and cooking methods. At current rates of growth, healthcare costs are projected to consume up to 22-24% of our nation's entire economy by 2017 (now at 23%!). Our opinion of causes of the current state of health decline in the US are the following trends: 1) an over-processed, genetically modified, degerminated, and micro-nutrient-deficient food supply; 2) chronic semi-dehydration coupled with dramatic increases in caffeine intake; 3) increased environmental toxins; 4) sedentary lifestyles and sleep disorders, 5) dramatically increased drug and alcohol addictions; and 6) a diet that is largely microwaved. This monograph explores why health conscientious families and individuals will want to refrain from microwaving, even for warming of their food.

Two Schools of Thought

Today, there are essentially two schools of thought on the current health scene in the US. On one side are those who argue that microwaving is the best cooking method ever, that GMOs are healthy for you, including high fructose corn syrup (HFCS), that high caffeine is essentially harmless, the problem with GMO-infused glutens are a non-topic, and there's not a dime's worth of difference between synthetic nutrients and those occurring naturally and organically. The other camp, which is growing steadily, is moving away from microwaving, using instead more fresh fruits and vegetables, convection, steaming, grilling, crockpot, etc. as preferred cooking methods; organic nutrition, hydration, moderation in caffeine, and abstinence from anything, like those extra glutens, tobacco, drugs, alcohol, etc. that are harmful to human health.

Empirical evidence is overwhelmingly on the side of the latter camp as we witness diabetes mellitus, neuropathies, CVD (including hypertension), arthritis, and most cancers resolve dramatically when eating more organically, hydrating, chelating, etc. Sleep disorders are resolved and infections and injuries heal faster. Yet the controversy still rages on, with the "official consensus" judging those of us who espouse natural and organic as complete heretics, at best.

On the pro-microwaving/GMO/synthetic side, billions in government and vested interest dollars are spent funding "research" that has been designed with short timelines, closed systems analysis, and which often fails to recognize biological factors. Meanwhile, the humble camp of scientists and practitioners on the natural/organic side receive practically no such funding, while conducting much smaller but more revealing studies than the well-heeled crowd. Let's review what the humble camp has to say on the matter—and then the reader can decide who is correct on the salient question of microwaving food.

Health Consequences of Microwaving

First, microwaving reportedly alters and destroys amino acids and covalent bonds of DNA in the food, the building blocks of life (i.e. the "microwave effect"—see http://www.rfsafe.com/archive/research/rf_hazards/dna_damage/microwave_effect.htm for a more complete treatment of this topic). In one study it was suggested that during microwaving that certain amino acids were converted into their carcinogenic and toxic d-isomer cousins. Nothing live survives microwaving, save some dreadful salmonella and e Coli bacteria. This causes one's immune system to produce *pro-inflammatory cytokines* that bring inflammation and the conditions that arise from inflammation and acidosis (perhaps 80% of all chronic disease results from inflammation!).

If you are wondering how this affects an otherwise healthy individual, look at your before/after changes in C-reactive protein scores (an inflammatory measure), triglycerides, and A1C scores (a hemoglobin/oxygen measure) in clinical blood tests when refraining from microwaving. The results can be quite stunning, as will be your overall health state.

The pH Cascade View of Food-to-Nutrition Synthesis & the KREB's Cycle without Microwaving

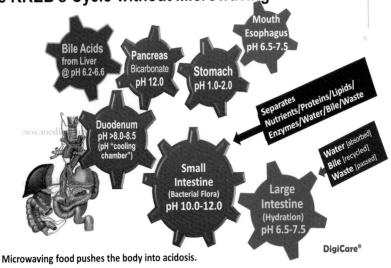

Microwaving food pushes the body into acidosis.

DigiCare®

Microwaving food also causes complex carbohydrates to be converted into simpler carbohydrates, which can *spike one's blood sugar, raise triglycerides,* and secrete too much fat-preserving *insulin,* while shutting off fat-burning *glycogen.* The result is *hyperinsulinemia,* arguably the biggest driver behind the obesity and diabetes pandemics in the United States today.

Only *synthetic nutrition* survives intact during microwaving, because organic nutrition complexes soon become *inorganic.* As mentioned above, the violent "microwave effect" on the DNA can make food "foreign" to the human digestive and immunological system, taking longer to digest and increasing allergies, in general. For certain, the body knows the difference between microwaved food and that prepared by other means, as evidenced by exploding rates of metabolic and digestive disorders seen in microwave-using consumers.

Because microwaved food must be reconstructed by the body by borrowing amino acids and enzymes, it can cause corresponding amino acid depletions in the precursors for **serotonin** (mood control), **melatonin** (sleep/wake cycle), and **dopamine** (motor control and tremor). These hormonal interruptions are increasingly evidenced by rising levels of abnormalities, such as depression, anxiety, sleep disorders, and tremor. Serotonin's *main* role is in food-to-nutrition synthesis and to aid in facilitating *glucagon and insulin* secretions. The disruption of serotonin, therefore, causes nutritional and metabolic abnormalities, including a rise in sugars being converted into triglycerides in the liver.

This is why SSRI and other anti-depressants actually *cause* diabetes and weight gain—since they also distort the prominent role of serotonin *without rectifying the real underlying causes of the depression for which they were prescribed.*

Further, we find that microwaved food requires the body to spend an extra 2-3 hours to digest food compared to optimally prepared meals. As mentioned above, that is because the body's immune system essentially suspends the food-to-nutrition synthesis functions while sorting out what has been ingested. This, in turn, can cascade into *acid reflux* (because the pyloric sphincter will not open until the pancreas has done its work), interruption of the *citric acid cycle in the liver*, elevated triglycerides and LDL cholesterol, and chronic conditions like *Irritable Bowel Syndrome* (IBS), etc.

Others have suggested that cooking meat in the microwave oven causes it to go into a kind of "rotting" process through destruction of nucleoproteins. This, in turn, causes the digested (and especially undigested) meat proteins to breakdown into cytotoxins and uric acid, setting off even more chronic disease. Metal and plastics are often added to packaged microwaved foods to simulate conventional cooking. While the altered taste and texture may fool *you*, it does not fool *your immune system*. Plus, these foods are loaded with gluten-infused GMO wheat!

Likewise, pets' health degrades substantially when eating from microwaved food, developing serious candida yeast and other disorders. Many veterinarian physicians are concerned about pets being fed the same over-processed, synthetically fortified, and degerminated microwaved foods their owners eat. For such increases risks of cancer and other human-like conditions in pets!

Of great concern, also, is that baby formulae and/or Mother's milk heated in plastic bottles in the microwave has been found to be unsafe for babies. Furthermore, dangerous levels of Bisphenol A (BPAs) found in today's microwavable food packaging have been linked to cancer, developmental disorders, diabetes, early puberty, and obesity in children. Some state health departments warn the public of these potential dangers.

In addition, every safety manual on warming of human blood for transfusions that we have examined says never use a microwave to warm the blood. This quiet affirmation that microwaving of blood is dangerous reinforces the thesis of the "microwave effect" even if it cannot be fully explained by sci-

Preparing Food for a Healthier Lifestyle

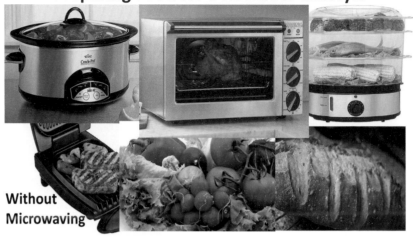

Without Microwaving

entists—many know it exists.

Before many governments clamped down and forbade further studies on safety of microwaving food, many independent studies reported what has been called "microwave sickness" in the literature: headache, dizziness, eye pain, sleeplessness, irritability, anxiety, stomach pain, nervous tension, inability to concentrate, hair loss, appendicitis, cataracts, sterility, and cancer. Many microwave ovens in use today reportedly leak radiation as a result of defective doors and insulation, especially as the over gets older.

Chronic and long-lasting symptoms from using microwave ovens have also been reported variously as adrenal exhaustion, ischemic heart disease, increased cancer cell formation, and long-term digestive disorders. Gradual breakdown of elimination systems in the body.

More importantly, as an adjunct to every good health program, are some guidelines on cooking:
- **Use a convection oven in place of microwaving for convenience and for safer cooking**
- **Eat a diet comprised of at least 50% fresh fruits and vegetables, non-GMO whole grains, and nuts**

- Steam vegetables when needed, *never* boil them—if one must cook on stovetop, use as little water as possible over low heat
- Use extra virgin olive oil and butter; avoid canola oil and other plasticized or over processed oils-avoid canola and other plasticized oils like the plague.
- Insist that restaurants not microwave or warm your food in a microwave—this is common in some restaurants like Chile's, Outback, and other high-volume chains.
- Reduce or eliminate caffeinated drinks; drink water
- Avoid GMO high fructose corn syrup and artificial sweeteners (Stevia is both safe and organic)

Note: Monographs by Dr. Chartrand cover hundreds of topics explaining how one may benefit from adult stem cell healing with cutting edge treatment approaches. For more information, contact: DigiCare Behavioral Research, 820 W. Cottonwood Lane, Suite #6, Casa Grande, AZ 85122, (520)509-6380.

References & Resources

Chartrand, MS, (2014), *How to Raise Your Body's pH,* Casa Grande, AZ: DigiCare Behavioral Research.

Chartrand, MS (2013). *Introducing Dr. Mitochondria*, (DVD Version) Casa Grande, AZ: DigiCare Behavioral Research.

Davis DR (February 1, 2009). "Declining fruit and vegetable nutrient composition: What is the evidence?" *American Society of Horticultural Science*

George DF, Bilek MM, and McKenzie DR (2010). Non-thermal effects in the microwave induced unfolding of proteins observed by chaperone binding.

Havas M (2012). "DECT phone affects the heart!"

Health effects of microwave radiation (Western view). "History of microwave ovens" *Green Health Watch*, undated.

Kakita Y, Kashige N, Murata K, Kuroiwa A, Funatsu M and Watanabe K. "Inactivation of Lactobacillus bacteriophage PL-

1 by microwave irradiation"
Kidmose U and Kaack K. Acta Agriculturae Scandinavica B
1999:49(2):110-117
Lee L. (12/9/1989). "Health effects of microwave radiation-
microwave ovens," *Lancet*
FDA (undated). "Microwave oven radiation," U.S. Food and Drug
Administration
Microwave oven and microwave cooking overview," Powerwatch
Microwave ovens: A danger to your health?" (January 26, 2010)
Nutritional and Physical Regeneration
Penn State U (2002). "DNA and the microwave effect", http://
www.rfsafe.com/archive/research/rf_hazards/dna_damage/
microwave_effect.htm.
Quan R, et al. (2012). "Effects of microwave radiation on anti-
infective factors in human milk," *Pediatrics 89*(4 part I):667-
669
Rust S and Kissinger M (November 15, 2008). "BPA leaches from
'safe' products" *Journal Sentinel Online.*
Sage C. "Reported biological effects from radiofrequency non-
ionizing radiation" Wave-Guide.org
Song K and Milner J A. (2001). "The influence of heating on the
anticancer properties of garlic," *Journal of Nutrition 2001; 131*
(3S):1054S-57S
Thomas W. (2013). "Cooked" *Alive.com*
Vallejo F, Tomas-Barberan FA, Garcia-Viguera C (2010).
"Phenolic compound contents in edible parts of broccoli inflo-
rescences after domestic cooking"
Villablanca E (December 19, 2007) "Ionizing and non-ionizing
radiation: Their difference and possible health consequences.

V

Overcoming Acid Reflux:
Righting what's Upside Down

Introduction: *If I was speaking to a room full of adults and asked those who suffer from acid reflux to raise their hands, about a third of the hands would reach for the sky. If I was to ask them if the problem is too much or too little acid, like a Gregorian chant I would hear "too much". And my reply would be, "Oh, really? Welcome to the Twilight Zone." For in today's dietary world, too little, not too much acid is the problem for at least 95% of sufferers of the alphabet soup of GERD/GORD/ GRD (gastroesophageal/ gastro-oesophageal/ gastric reflux disease). Lost in the world of microwaved, genetically modified, synthetically fortified, degerminated, chemically preserved, and artificially colored & flavored food, is that nothing about most of the recent modifications to the food we eat is good for the human body. Our children are not developing, as increasingly more and more suffer from developmental disorders, from increased rates of breathing and allergy disorders to skyrocketing increases in learning and behavioral disorders. Even our pets die an early death when fed what we eat, especially if it has been microwaved. So, now we ask those who raised their hands to read on. Learn how to change your life—the SIRCLE® Method way!*

Not *Enough* Acid, You Say?

Yes, you see, the *healthy* stomach has an acid-alkaline balance of pH 1.2-2.0 (on a logarithmic scale of 1.0-14.0). It was meant to be a veritable caldron of acid to: **1)** create an "acid barrier" to kill the bacteria & viruses (and parasites) we ingest each day, without which we would become ill with the slight-

43

est amount of same (stomach flu, anyone?), **2)** help us absorb vital nutrients, such as iron, copper, zinc, calcium, folic acid, B-12, and various proteins, and **3)** break down food components into a fine puree (created from quantities of HCL, citric acid, pepsin, and bicarbonate) so that it can emptied through a pencil-sized opening at the pyloric sphincter into the duodenum within about 25-minutes of entering the stomach. In the duodenum, bile acids are sprayed onto fatty lipids to maximize HDL, minimize LDL for their specialized purposes in your body. When food reaches the small intestine, differentiation then occurs to sort out energy, nutrients, and waste (food-to-nutrition synthesis) until we achieve that balanced state called *homeostasis.*

Description of the Reflux Cascade
The *reality* is that today's modern stomach boasts a puny

Key Player: The Pancreas

I. The exocrine pancreas:

A. Secretes digestive enzymes through ducts in response to the duodenal hormone *cholecystokini* *(CCK)* for digestion of fats, starches, and proteins

B. Secretes *bicarbonate* solution in response to the duodenal hormone *secretin* to neutralize acids entering the small intestine

II. The endocrine pancreas:
A. After digested fats and starches enter the blood stream, secretes the hormones *insulin* and *glucagc* into bloodstream as needed

B. Secretes somatostatin, which acts as the "brak on hormones (insulin and glucagon) as needed by cells of the body

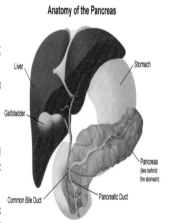
Anatomy of the Pancreas

Liver
Stomach
Gallbladder
Pancreas (les behind the stomach)
Common Bile Duct
Pancreatic Duct

pH 3.0, acidic enough to scar the esophagus during reflux events, but not nearly acidic enough to kill bacteria, absorb nutrients, and breakdown half-chewed, over-processed nutrient-starved "food".

In truth, since the majority of illness in the US today is comprised of acid-based conditions (poor digestion, IBS, Crohn's disease, Celiac disease, hypertriglyceridemia, alkaline liver, diabetes type 2, neuropathy, arthritis, cancer, etc.). *Hydrochloria,* or low stomach acids, contributes mightily to these conditions, and causes many sufferers to also suffer *frequent food poisoning* because of lack of acid barrier. These episodes are too often mistaken for "stomach flu", which is a really rare form of flu, indeed!

The reason so many think they have *too much* stomach acid is because the food stays in their stomach for 2-4 hours or more and never really digests. This causes a "stenosis" of the duodenum, causing the food to reflux back up into the esophagus, especially when lying down. As stated earlier, the acid & partly broken down food is strong enough to burn the esophagus, even the pharynx/larynx, yet it is nowhere near acidic enough to break down the food enough so that nutrition can be extracted by the time is reaches the upper intestine.

Righting what's Upside Down

As in all chronic conditions, the objectives are to repair unhealed injuries, make sure infections and inflammatory states

Why acid reflux medications are among the most dangerous of <u>long-term</u> medications

- **Cause significant Bone Loss & Fractures**
- **Chronic & Acute Anemia**
- **Block B-Vitamins, especially B-12**
- **Contribute to Neuropathy**
- **Cognitive Disorders/Alzheimer disease**
- **Chronic Bronchitis/ Pneumonia**
- **Chronic Colitis & Colon Cancer**
- **Hypothyroidism/Thyroid Disorders**
- **Hypertension, Cardiovascular Disease**
- **...and More!** (ex: contributes to tumor growth)

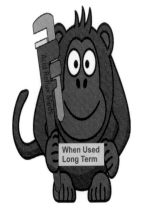

45

are corrected, and restore the biomarkers of cellular acid-alkaline balance to pH 7.45, oxygen to 99-100%, A1C below 5.0, CRP below 1.0, Gelactin-3 below 17.1%, electrolytes in perfect balance, and cartilage, bone, and cardiovascular state is normalized. These markers tell us how close to "homeostasis" we have come with diet and lifestyle.

Now, let's set upright what has turned our lives upside down by observing a few simple but important rules:

1. **No more microwaving**, not even to warm up your food. Read the labels, avoiding Aspartame (in sugar-free gum and most diet sodas), MSG, high fructose, bromulated vegetable oil, canola oil, and, as much as possible, avoid GMOs, caffeinated drinks, and foods with gluten.

2. **Start all meals with fresh vegetables and fruits *before* eating any meat;** eating meat sparingly. Drink no more than 1/2 glass of anything during the meal—finishing the remainder at the end of the meal.

3. **Chew your food to a paste,** mixing saliva thoroughly before swallowing. This neutralizes acids and prepares the food for quick digestion. It also brings earlier satiation, so you will less inclined to overeat. Lack of satiation is the #1 reason for weight gain.

4. **Use 1-2 drops of doTerra essential oil combination Digestzyn in 3-4 oz. of water** before every meal until your acid reflux is no more. Then, as prophylaxis, once every few days or when digestion occurs.

5. **Take (1) or (2) Apple Cider Vinegar Capsules** at the start of at least two meals per day for 30 days, overlapping with your acid reflux meds by about a week. Then, as you phase out your reflux meds, you will find you will digest your food better and overcoming the deficiencies caused by the reflux medications.

6. **Eat at least 3 hours before retiring for bed.** Never eat and lie down right afterward, unless you don't mind indigestion! In fact, avoid eating for at least 3 hours at a

stretch so that your body can regain its pH and digestive efficiency. It takes the pancreas three hours just to make enough bicarbonate to open the duodenum for the next meal.

7. **The best reflux "quick remedy" is ionized alkaline water.** It is faster, at lower cost, and will allow you to regain your health!

8. **To help wean off acid reflux meds, use an essential oil combination called Digestzen,** (1) drop in 4 oz. of water just before breakfast and dinner for as long as it takes to reset your metabolism. A distant second to using Digestzen is (1) apple cider vinegar capsules about 15 minutes before each meal until digestion is back to normal.

Note: Monographs by Dr. Chartrand cover hundreds of topics explaining how one may benefit from adult stem cell healing with cutting edge treatment approaches. For more information, contact: DigiCare Behavioral Research, 820 W. Cottonwood Lane, Suite #6, Casa Grande, AZ 85122, (520)509-6380.

More Resources

Chartrand, M.S. (2013). How to Raise Your Body's pH & Overcome Chronic Disease. Casa Grande, AZ: DigiCare Behavioral Research.

Hofmann, A., and Mysels, K. (1992). Bile acid solubility and precipitation in vitro and in vivo: the role of conjugation, pH, and Ca2+ ions. Journal of Lipid Research. http://www.jlr.org/content/33/5/617.full.pdf

Thirteen Foods That Fight Acid Reflux (2013). http://www.health.com/health/gallery/0,,20440834,00.html

Tips for Overcoming GERD (2013). http://www.gibay.com/articles/houston-acid-reflux-3-tips-to-overcoming-gerd.html.

VI

HIGH FRUCTOSE CORN SYRUP:
Recipe for Obesity, Heart Disease & Diabetes Type 2

Introduction: It is well known that major changes in the US food supply have contributed mightily to the chronic disease pandemics that are unique to our nation. Less recognized, however, is that, until the food companies start using healthier sweeteners like Stevia and organic cane sugar (hopefully half and half), only consumers can change this alarming scenario: by avoiding as much as possible that which is contributing 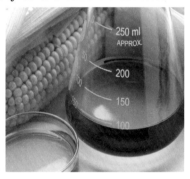 to their ill health, choosing instead dietary options that promise significantly greater health. *Hence, consumers hold the power to bring about the badly needed changes, if they will.* Every new entrant into the health fold adds to the strength of those who are already there. Then, the merchants of food will follow suit, gingerly so.

HFCS: Dominant "Added Sugar" to Food Supply

High Fructose Corn Syrup (HFCS) is a concentrated genetically-modified organism (GMO) processed from GMO corn, and used as the predominant sweetener in nearly all popular soft drinks, candies, baked goods, and just about every type of commercially processed food (Barrett, 2012). It is by far the most ubiquitous GMO out there, and there are very few people in the US whose diet is not dominated by it.

While we do not suggest that all things bad in health lay at the doorstep of HFCS, when one adds the other trends, such as microwaving of food (killing amino acids), high caffeine intake (leading to adrenal depletion and acidosis), and a food supply that is degerminated, irradiated, synthetically fortified, and absent of nearly all micro nutrients, HFCS becomes one more major trend that consumers need to avoid en masse, if they wish to see it taken back out of the food supply.

Alters Human Metabolism through Fast Absorption

Today, we have an epidemic of diabetes type 2 sweeping the United States—with more than 81 million pre-diabetics and 39 million diabetics (counting undiagnosed cases). Obesity and cardiovascular disease continue to skyrocket as a result. At this time it appears that the single largest contributing factor is the universal addition of HFCS sugars to the nation's food supply. It's much smaller molecular size and simpler chemistry causes it to enter the bloodstream without converting first to glucose and fructose—as more natural sugars do—and converts quickly to fat.

Processed (Dead) vs Natural (Live) Foods
Microwave/Processed Foods vs Fresh/Slow-Cooked Foods

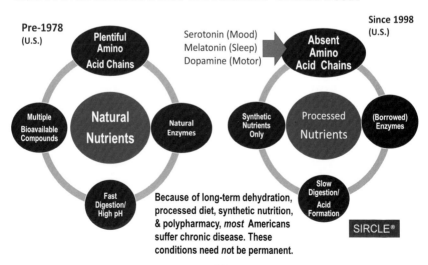

Pre-1978 (U.S.) — Plentiful Amino Acid Chains — Serotonin (Mood) Melatonin (Sleep) Dopamine (Motor) — Since 1998 (U.S.) — Absent Amino Acid Chains

Multiple Bioavailable Compounds — **Natural Nutrients** — Natural Enzymes — Synthetic Nutrients Only — Processed Nutrients — (Borrowed) Enzymes

Fast Digestion/ High pH — Slow Digestion/ Acid Formation

Because of long-term dehydration, processed diet, synthetic nutrition, & polypharmacy, *most* Americans suffer chronic disease. These conditions need *not* be permanent.

SIRCLE®

HFCS has also been implicated in turning off the cell signaling process, so that the body is unable to decide what nutrients your body needs. This, in turn, leads to faster weight gain and cardiovascular disease. A recent study at UC Davis demonstrated increased fat deposits around the heart and in the abdominal cavity, raising triglycerides in the liver, and increasing insulin resistance in research subjects as a result of HFCS ingestion compared to controls that were given standard sugars. Another study at UCLA found HFCS reduced memory and learning function.

Aggressive media advertising by the Corn Refiners Association (CRA) has attempted to counter results from these independent studies by claiming that HFCS is as natural as standard sugars. But many things that are adverse to human health are "natural", especially when genetically modified to make the food cheaper, more plentiful, and requiring less fertilization and water to produce.

Princeton Study Confirmation

One of my colleagues in a 2010 study at Princeton studied the differences in food additive sweeteners. Now this study was on rats, but don't let that put you off. Better them than you, right? I will quote what they reported in a news release:

"Some people have claimed that high fructose corn syrup is no different than other sweeteners when it comes to weight gain and obesity, but our results make it clear this just isn't true, at least under the conditions of our tests...When rats are drinking high-fructose corn syrup at levels well below those in soda pop, they're becoming obese—every single one of them, across the board. Even when rats are fed a high fat diet, you don't see this; [in high fat diets] they don't all gain extra weight."

Guidelines for a "Healthy" Diet?

One of the challenges with which Americans are faced today is the federal dietary guidelines that walk the tightrope between trying to promote a healthy population and keeping vested interests happy. In their suggested guidelines, the Food & Nutrition Board (FNB) of the National Academy of Sciences maintains that synthetic nutrition and bioavailable organic nutrition are equals, and that all commercially available added sugars are the same. In fact, even the predominant non-sugar sweeteners—Aspartame, NutraSweet®, Saccharin, all shown dangerous—and the manifold neurotoxic chemicals & heavy metals in processed foods are anything but safe for human consumption.

Collins and Collins (2006), the authors of the celebrated *The China Study*, portrayed the absurdity of federal guidelines by showing what one could eat in one day and still ostensibly stay within the guidelines.

☐ **FOR BREAKFAST:** (1) cup HFCS Fruit Loops, (1) cup skim milk, (1) package of HFCS M&Ms, and a synthetic multiple vitamin and fiber.
☐ **FOR LUNCH:** (1) Grilled cheeseburger
☐ **FOR DINNER:** (3) slices of pepperoni pizza, (1) 16 oz. HFCS soda, and (1) HFCS Archway cookie.

It goes without saying, it is time to get over our diabetes, overweight, memory, and cardiovascular problems. That means reading the labels of everything your family consumes and avoiding that which does not provide their optimum health. High fructose, a highly concentrated, genetically, and extremely cheap added sweetener is one of the most important ingredients to especially avoid and minimize as much as possible. The body *does* know the difference.

Note: Monographs by Dr. Chartrand cover hundreds of topics explaining how one may benefit from adult stem cell healing with cutting edge treatment approaches. For more information, contact: DigiCare Behavioral Research, 820

W. Cottonwood Lane, Suite #6, Casa Grande, AZ 85122, (520)509-6380.

FOR FURTHER STUDY

Chaitowitz, S. (2004). *Court rules against USDA's secrecy and failure to disclose conflict of interest in setting nutrition policies.* Physicians Committee for Responsible Nutrition, http://pcrm.org/news/health001002.html.

Chartrand, M. (2012). Dr. Mitochondria & You: How to Get Well (from whatever ails you). Consumer DVD. Casa Grande, AZ: DigiCare® Behavioral Research

Collins, T.C., and Collins, T.M. (2006). *The China Study.* Dallas: BenBella Books, Inc., ISBN 1-932100-66-0.

Food & Nutrition Board, and Institute of Medicine (2010). "Dietary reference intakes for energy, carbohydrates, fiber, fat, fatty acids, cholesterol, protein, and amino acids," Washington, DC: The National Academy Press.

Gucciardia, A. (2012). Report on the UCLA High Fructose Corn Syrup Memory Study. http://naturalsociety.com/high-fructose-corn-syrup-damages-learning-abilities-memory/

Gucciardia, A. (2012). Report on the UC-Davis High Fructose Corn Syrup Study. http://www.naturalnews.com/study.html.

Princeton University (2010). A Sweet Problem: Princeton researchers find that high-frustose corn syrup prompts considerably more weight gain. http://www.princeton.edu/main/newsarchive/S26/91/22K07/.

VII
Understanding Bone Loss
Osteoarthritis-Osteopenia-Osteoporosis & Other Bone Disorders

Introduction: *During their lifetimes, at least half of those over age 50 will be at risk of developing osteoporosis. When we speak of bone loss we are primarily speaking of three diagnostic stages: Osteoarthritis (1-2% loss per annum), Osteopenia (3% per annum), and Osteoporosis (4-5%+ per annum) that are caused almost entirely by diet, hydration, lifestyle, medications, and environmental stressors. Rather than attacking un-*

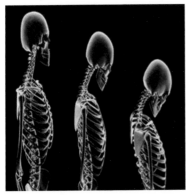

derlying causes in each case, it has become expedient in the business of healthcare to ignore those and go instead for over-medicalized symptoms, false models of healing, and erroneous data in support of a business model that leaves affected patients worse off than if they did nothing. The truth is, if one truly desires to restore good bone health they will start by restoring good health first and attacking head -on the utterly avoidable and underlying causes that caused their debilitative state in the first place.

Osteoblasts vs Osteoclasts Human bones are highly vascularized and mineralized tissues that are constantly being shaped and developed by cells called *osteoblasts* and torn down and resorbed by cells called *osteoclasts*. Recent research confirms that throughout one's lifespan it is osteoblast activity that controls and dictates osteoclast activity as long as the body receives the nutrients it requires to maintain homeostasis. Growing children, for instance, have a far greater abundance of osteoblasts than of osteoclasts. By the time they reach young adulthood (at about age 26 for men, 22 for women) osteoclasts increase while osteoblasts slow down. Even so, humans of any age can increase osteoblast activity and slow the formation of osteoclasts through weight bearing exercise and other methods. The problem of bone shrinkage

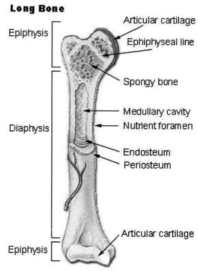

Long Bone
Epiphysis
Articular cartilage
Ephiphyseal line
Spongy bone
Diaphysis
Medullary cavity
Nutrient foramen
Endosteum
Periosteum
Articular cartilage
Epiphysis

and decline in strength presents most often in health states involving:

☐ **Sedentary Lifestyle**, making weight bearing exercise a frontline defense against bone loss for everyone.

☐ **Acidosis** (low cellular pH), from a diet that is microwaved, nutritionally lacking, genetically modified, degerminated, irradiated, laden with toxins & over-processed.

☐ **Chronic dehydration** from too much caffeine and high fructose corn syrup (a highly concentrated GMO sweetener) and not enough water.

☐ **Lacking in calcium** that is live, ionically charged, as well as phosphorus, magnesium, boron, and other minerals comprised in human bones. On the other hand, commercially available calcium is inert calcium that causes atherosclerosis, kidney stones, bone spurs, cataracts, and bone loss!

☐ **Taking prescription medications**, especially acid reflux meds, NSAIDs, osteoporosis meds, and steroids over the long term. These and more interfere with osteoblast activity and weaken immunology.

☐ **Unhealed injuries** and deterioration of the spine, such as compression fractures (>50% of the US adult population), spinal stenosis, kyphosis, and scoliosis. These cause even more rapid loss of bone mass.

☐ **Subclinical infections:** tooth and gum sepsis, around artificial joints, keratosis obturans, kidney and bladder infections, neuropathies, and osteomyelitis as a result of injuries and/or shock to the bones.

☐ **Heavy metal accumulations:** lead, mercury, cadmium, arsenic, formaldehyde, cyanide, etc. found in the drinking water, fresh foods, cosmetics, paints, fuels, and a host of commonly used products.

☐ **Lifestyle Substances–** Smoking, alcohol, excess coffee, marijuana, opium (including opiate pain killers), diet sodas, caffeine drinks.

Osteoporosis Meds Fraught with Risks

Independent researchers are deeply concerned that poorly designed and self-serving studies and fudged numbers have sold a bill of goods to physicians and consumers on the long-term efficacy of alendronate, etidronate, risedronate, bisphosphonate, and zoleronic acid drugs (Fosamax, Boniva, Reclast, etc.). Overprescribing these drugs has brought unfathomable suffering in the form of: doubled cancer risk, ulcers of the esophagus, upper GI irritation, fractures of the femur, low blood calcium, skin rash, joint pain, jaw bone decay, increased parathyroid hormone secretions, and early death.

Types of Bone Disorders

Common Disorders
• Osteoarthritis
• Osteopenia
• Osteoporosis
• Spinal Stenosis
• Compression Fractures
• Rheumatoid Arthritis ◀

Less Common Disorders
• Ankylosing Spondylitis
• Paget's Disease
• Osteogenesis Imperfecta
• Fibrodysplasia Ossificans Progressiva
• More than 6,000 others!

Nearly always RA is caused by untreated infection or sepsis
somewhere in the body, usually in the head and neck area.

These drugs simply make the periosteum and teeth brittle, fill the bones with dead bone cells (osteoclasts), and after five years' use, spontaneous fractures become even *more* lethal. Filling the bones with dead cells makes bone density test results look good in x-ray, but do nothing to improve the bones!

Remediation and Treatment

Here are some of the treatment aspects that must be addressed before medication or surgery should be considered:

Diet: Stop microwaving, eat at least 50% of your diet in fresh fruits and vegetables. Avoid GMO high fructose corn syrup and *all* (processed) artificial sweeteners. Use Extra Virgin Olive Oil, avoid Canola Oil.

Targeted Nutrition: Utilization of Microcrystalline Hydroxyapatite Compound (MCHC), etc.; avoid synthetic vitamins/inert minerals.

Hydration: Drink filtered, ionized, alkalized water. Avoid/reduce caffeine.

Heavy Metals: Chelate heavy metals with CardioFlow.

Toxins, Medications: As biomarkers improve, with your doctor's guidance, wean off medications that cause bone loss and destruction, such as all acid reflux medications, long-term steroids, and osteoporosis medications. Refrain from using tobacco, alcohol, recreational drugs.

Spinal & Accumulated Injuries: All injuries need to be addressed. As the spine & injuries heal, most neuropathies resolve and bone mass flourishes. Deep Cold Laser, Far Infrared, Medical Massage, AromaTouch®, Neuromuscular Retraining, Chiropractics, Dentistry, etc. become the healing modalities of choice over surgical manipulation, most certainly in cases of degeneration.

Subclinical Infections: Usually found in the jaw and teeth, ear, lungs, artificial joints, feet & intestines. Such are a major cause of inflammation.

Note: Monographs by Dr. Chartrand cover hundreds of top-

ics explaining how one may benefit from adult stem cell healing with cutting edge treatment approaches. For more information, contact: DigiCare Behavioral Research, 820 W. Cottonwood Lane, Suite #6, Casa Grande, AZ 85122, (520)509-6380.

Resources for Further Study

Brown, S.E. (2014). Osteoporosis risks vs benefits of osteoporosis drugs—spinning the numbers. http://www.betterbones.com/osteoporosis/risks-benefits.aspx.

Chartrand, MS (2013). *Introducing Dr. Mitochondria*, CG, AZ: DigiCare Behavioral Research.

Clinical Summary (2014). Evaluation of Nutritional Support with Concentrated Microcrystalline Hydroxyapatite Concentrate. https://nutri-dyn.com/images/LinkedCases/MET1248.pdf

Goldschmidt, V. (2014). *Is Sugar Toxic for Your Bones?* http://saveourbones.com/is-sugar-toxic-for-your-bones/.

Lee L. (1989). "Health effects of microwave radiation-microwave ovens," *Lancet*

Pines, A., Raafat, H., Lynn, A.H., Whittington, J. (1984). Clinical trial of microcrystalline hydroxyapatite compound in the prevention of osteoporosis due to corticosteroid therapy. *Current Medical Research Opinions*, 8(10):734-42.

Rust & Kissinger (2008). "BPA leaches from 'safe' products" *Journal Sentinel Online*.

Villablanca E (December 19, 2007) "Ionizing and non-ionizing radiation: Their difference and possible health consequences.

Yasuda, H. (2012). New roles of osteoblasts in osteoclast differentiation. http://www.wjgnet.com/2218-5836/pdf/v3/i11/175.pdf.

VIII

CHRONIC FATIGUE SYNDROME
Roadmap to Diabetes Mellitus II, Osteoarthritis, Cardiovascular Disease, Cancer and Early Aging

Introduction: *For good or bad, one's mind is the master over their body. The mind decides what food and drink to give the body, and, to some extent, how it will be digested. It decides if and when one sleeps—and for how long. It decides whether to get up and exercise, work, or play. The mind has attitude and intent, and causes hormones to secrete, synapses to fire away, and whether little or big things will disrupt one's life. And, conversely, the mind can make one's life serene and tranquil even in the midst of extreme deprivation and chaos. One's mind, in short, decides whether to be well or not, happy or sad, or angry or contented, and whether one will get up on his or her own hind-legs, take one's health by the horns, and make it a smashing success story against all odds...If one will do it!*

Chronic Fatigue Syndrome Defined

From the US Centers of Disease Control (CDC) comes, *"Chronic fatigue syndrome, or CFS, is a debilitating and complex disorder characterized by profound fatigue that is not improved by bed rest and that may be worsened by physical or mental activity. Symptoms affect several body systems and may include weakness, muscle pain, impaired memory and/or mental concentration, and insomnia, which can result in reduced participation in daily activities."*

In Behavioral Medicine, CFS represents a culmination of causal factors, such as lack of restorative sleep, lack of exercise, too much caffeine, long-term micronutrient deficiencies, chronic dehydration, heavy metal accumulations, unresolved infections and injuries, and too many prescription medications.

Misdiagnosis/Mistreatment of CFS Common

One reason that CFS is so often misdiagnosed is because the most prominent symptomatic manifestations garner all of the attention under today's treatment practices. Because the current system has *overmedicalized* symptoms as if they are pathologies, ignoring the more salient underlying causes, CFS presents a mass of confusion to the world of medical diagnostics. Some CFS, for instance, is misdiagnosed as **fibromyalgia**, because fibromyalgia, inflamed joints, and muscle pain are so similar in symptomology. Certainly, the pain effects can be identical, even if the contributing factors are not.

Adrenal depletion is a common component of CFS, and is often misdiagnosed, because adrenal glands are so overburdened from too much caffeine, or from heavy metals, toxic food additives, or high quantities of GMO high fructose corn syrup (the most common sweetener in the US food supply). These can evoke symptoms of depression and/or anxiety, as well. Instead of insisting that CFS patients reduce caffeine and high fructose intake, dangerous SSRI/SNRI antidepressants or neuroleptic medication are prescribed like candy, leaving the underlying problem raging on.

Many **prescription medications**, especially where adverse side effects compound, cause an extraordinarily high number of cases of CFS in the US. **Opioid pain killers** are so common in the US that Americans consume over 80% of the world's medical grade opium, including heroin, unwittingly trapping tens of millions of Americans in inescapable addictions. Now, America finds

CHRONIC FATIGUE SYNDROME:
[One of the Most Under-/Mis-diagnosed Chronic Conditions in the US]

Devastating tiredness/exhaustion > six months

Substantially interferes with work, play, social life

Forgetfulness, memory loss, difficulty concentrating

Features tender lymph nodes in neck and armpits, sore throat, without explanation

Chronic muscle/joint pain, persistent inflammation

One of the most common features is sleeplessness

Nearly always associated w/ neuropathy & acidosis

Depleted adrenals (usually from too much caffeine or meds)

itself with a **dangerous epidemic of heroin and opioid addictions,** precisely because of these utterly irresponsible treatment practices. Hence, more than twice as many Americans die every year from opioid overdose than die on our highways!

Complaints of **tender lymph nodes in the neck and armpits, sore throat, and low grade fever**—a common component in CFS—often arises from tooth and/or jaw sepsis trapped under crowns and root canals and rotted teeth. But who's paying attention? Many of these cascade into chronic allergies and upper respiratory distress. which get treated with health-robbing corticosteroids, NSAIDs, and overuse of antibiotics.

Profound Fatigue: Drugged Sleep is Not the Answer

A common underlying contributor of CFS is lack of restorative sleep. More than 60 million Americans take prescription medication "to help them sleep". But, in reality, medications do not lead to restorative sleep, and sufferers continue their downward descent to loss of DNA telomeres, and dramatically shortened DNA strands, loss of mitochondria—**in a nutshell: rapid aging**—because core problems are disregarded. From the illustration below, one can readily see why restorative sleep is so crucial for quality of life and longevity. Without it we die far younger than we should.

"But," we often hear, *"I can't sleep without the drugs".* Our answer is always, *"actually, you can't really sleep with them. Instead, you need to find and address the underlying causes that are keeping you from enjoying a good night's sleep."* But, alas, the system is fraught with extremely costly, self-perpetuating "half measures" that instead lead to...more...problems.

Current Practice Standards: Half Measures

Treatment courses typically used in CFS cases treat only symptoms. A quick review of the "temporary half measures", currently prescribed for CFS more often than not, are:

- **Anticonvulsants,** or anti-seizure medications, like Gabapentin (Neurontin) and Pregabalin, which are laden with damaging long-term side effects.

- **Overuse of corticosteroids and antibiotics** for extended periods of time, letting the "party roll on" while bone mass depletes, affected cartilage fails to regenerate, setting the stage for stroke, CVD, and cancer.

- **Opioid pain killers, and/or SSRI/SNRI Antidepressants and nerve deadeners**, which ruin the liver and compromise immunological functions, bring addiction and deadly withdrawal issues, and in the end, is *totally* ineffective at resolving the pain for which it was prescribed.

- **Non-steroidal anti-inflammatories (NSAIDS)**, whose main actions draw blood, oxygen, and essential nutrients away from the site of lesion and literally turn off one's natural immunological repair system.

- **Amphetamines, sedatives, tranquilizers, and neuroleptic medications**, ostensibly to help one to "sleep" and to "wake up" from the brain fog that is typically caused from taking too many medications.

Note: Until substances like caffeine, alcohol, tobacco, opioids and other harmful drugs are eliminated, along with GMO 24-chromosome gluten-laden wheat products, high fructose corn syrup, certain food additives, microwaved food and unnecessary medications, and the patient finally achieves drug-free sleep, little progress will be realized in cases of CFS.

Caution: It is imperative that individuals make no changes to their prescribed medication without professional guidance.

"Our Heroes": Mitochondria, ATP & Stem Cells

From Lin et al. (2010): *"The potential to heal once incurable degenerative diseases by regenerating cells that have failed or are about to fail is now within our grasp, thanks to the emergence of regenerative medicine using adult stem cells...Their potential to differentiate into cell types found in other tissues [such as cartilage] means they can travel to the site of damage, penetrate the damaged tissue, and then regenerate this tissue by a process called transdifferentiation."*

The SIRCLE® Method begins with discovery of all contributing factors in one's health profile, and mapping out a program that addresses each contributing factor via specialized core and adjunct modalities until the body is returned as closely as possible to optimal health. The principles for therapeutic approaches are laid down in solid science and innovation, making it the lowest cost route to full healing. Progress is measured by Case History and Biomarker changes.

Central to the SIRCLE® program is lengthening of DNA and their "bookends" called telomeres, raising cellular oxygen levels as close to 100% as possible, and achieving cellular pH to 7.45 (per the Kreb's cycle). Then, through stimulation of the mitochondria and its ATP production, biomarkers begin to dramatically improve within weeks and months, allowing formation of more adult stem cells, which are directed to the site(s) of lesion that are causing the pain and loss of function. Lost height is recovered as spinal discs are repaired and expanded to their original size, skin becomes thicker and smoother, circulation improves all over the body, as well as re-establishment of neural tissues and bone mass.

In CFS, each case is different, requiring different lengths of time and attention to achieve the desired results. But, in all cases, quality of life can be vastly improved, function can be restored, and life can be extended far beyond expectations. In other words, mind over matter starts with taking the bull by the horns and getting one's life back...with SIRCLE®!***

Note: Other Monographs by Dr. Chartrand cover various aspects of the SIRCLE® Method for a wide array of chronic conditions. Contact: DigiCare Behavioral Research, 820 W. Cottonwood Ln, Ste #6, Casa Grande, AZ 85122, (520)509-6380.

Resources for Further Study

American Psychological Association (2017). How to get a good night's sleep. Found at http://www.apa.org/topics/sleep/why.aspx.

Chakkalakal, JV, Jones, KM, Basson, MA, Brack, AS (2012). The Aged Niche Disrupts Stem Muscle Cell Quiescence. *Nature, 490*, 355-360.

Chartrand, M.S. (2017). Understanding Neuropathy: Fibromyalgia, Peripheral & Diabetic Neuropathy, Restless Legs, Chronic Numbness/Burning, etc., DigiCare Behavioral Research, Casa Grande, AZ.

Cleveland Clinic (2014). Center for Continuing Education. http://www.clevelandclinic.meded.com/medicalpubs/diseasemanagement/neurology/peripheral-neuropathy/.

Graedon, J. (2012). Surprising Gabapentin Side Effects. Found at https://www.peoplespharmacy.com/2012/05/26/gabapentin-side-effects/

Lee L. (1989). "Health effects of microwave radiation," *Lancet*

Lin, F. et. al. (2010). Lasers, stem cells, and COPD. Journal of Translational Medicine, 8:16, doi: 10.1186/1479-5876-8-16.

National Institutes of Health (2014). Stem Cell Information. http://stemcells.nih.gov/static re-sources/info/basics/StemCellBasics.pdf

National Institute of Neurological Disorders and Stroke. Peripheral Neuropathy Fact Sheet. http://www.ninds.nih.gov/disorders/peripheralneuropathy/detail_peripheralneuropathy.htm.

Right Diagnosis (2014). Myoclonic Jerks and Papilloedema. http://symptoms. rightdiagnosis.com/cosymptoms/myoclonic-jerking/papilloedema-desc-sall.htm

Rogerson, D., Rothenberg, R., and Marasco, W, (2007). Report: Adult Stem Cell Therapies. *Life Extension*, October, 2007.

United States Centers for Disease Control (2017). Defining Chronic Fatigue Syndrome. Found at (https://www.cdc.gov/cfs/index.html)

IX

Septic Dental Disorders:
Unrecognized Public Health Threat

Introduction: *Whether an abscessed tooth, a septic keratosis obturans in the ear canal, an appendicitis, or a septic ingrown toe-nail, a common immunological thread connects all of these conditions: they can communicate with each other and even reinforce each other, creating more serious life-threatening disease when not attended to on a timely basis. In this monograph, the author reviews the hidden dangers of dental infections that often go overlooked, sometimes for years.*

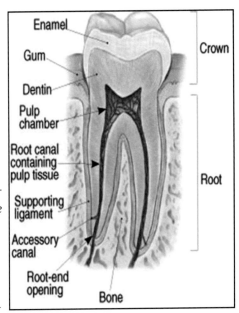

Tooth Sepsis Cascades to Other Disease if Left Untended

In scientific circles there is an ongoing debate over whether periodontal disease *causes* heart disease, or if it is just coincidental that the chance of heart disease doubles when one has periodontal disease. As a researcher, and Behavioral Medicine Consultant, my response is, since the most immunologically active sepsis in most people comes from the teeth and jaw, poor dental health equals poor heart health, to some degree. Here's what we see *routinely* in those with active periodontal disease: hypoxia (low oxygen with trapped CO2), low cellular <pH 7.0, spiked fasting blood sugar >120, and general body inflammation @ >1.0 CRP/>17.3 Gelactin-3 score. In a nutshell: *Not the picture of good heart health by a long shot.*

After taking care of the infection of periodontal disease, you may *still* not be totally out of the woods. That's because we find a certain subset of individuals who also have **Septic Keratosis Obturans** in the ear canal that developed during the time of the tooth sepsis—see my research monograph under this topic. Septic Keratosis Obturans, which appear to be growing rapidly in prevalence in the general population, are potentially lethal if allowed to follow their natural course without timely removal. Yet, almost always they are treated as if they are simple impacted earwax. However, they harbor nearly the same deadly bacterial colonies found in periodontal disease (i.e., anaerobic streptococci & pseudomonas, anaerobic Gram-negative bacilli, aspergillus favus, Enterobacter cloacae, etc.).

These bacteria can be harbored under crowns and root canals that elude x-ray inspection, in cavities where fillings have loosened or fallen out, and most certainly in cracked and/or abscessed teeth. Unflossed teeth harbor some of these bacteria, also. The body's immune response is to produce a proliferation of pro-inflammatory cytokines all over the body, and a rise in blood sugar. Sepsis in the teeth/jaw region has been implicated in cases of (partial listing):

Developing heart disease (via endocarditis, angina)
Clinical depression and anxiety (via cortical inflammation)
Upper intestinal infection (and chronic digestive disorders)
Neuropathy of the feet in diabetics (causing amputations)
Sepsis and inflammation around implanted prosthetics
Complicated Hypertension (atherosclerosis with inflammation)

Diabetes Mellitus Type 2 (in cases of uncontrollable or varying blood glucose)
Rheumatoid Arthritis
Kidney/Liver Failure
Pancreatitis/Gall Stones
"Walking Pneumonia"/Inhalant allergies
Increased food sensitivities

The truth is that, besides the loss of one's teeth in one fell swoop, there is also grave danger of cascading into far more serious disease elsewhere in the body when we ignore our dental health. The incidence of sepsis under crowns is skyrocketing today and, because these cannot be detected in x-rays, are often passed over.

Likewise, amalgam and composite fillings eventually shrink, and bacteria finds its way (all it takes is a few molecules of bacteria!) inside the tooth, or heaven help us, to the root of the tooth and to the underlying structure of the jaw.

These can go septic and start a cascade of other diseases in the body over time. For this reason, it is vital that one locates a dentist or oral surgeon who understands these disorders and is willing to look deeper than mere x-ray and visual inspection. Then, do what is necessary to correct the problem and keep your teeth in immaculate condition.

Otherwise, sepsis can be harbored in the mouth by simply not flossing daily, or from microscopic cracks in the teeth, and most especially around and below fillings and under crowns. Therefore, observation of good dental health habits and maintenance become imperative in preventing other more serious disease, and in living a life to one's full potential.

SIRCLE: Powerful Adjunct to Good Dental Health

As in all chronic conditions, the objectives are to repair unhealed injuries, make sure infections and inflammatory states are corrected, and restore the biomarkers of cellular acid-alkaline balance to pH 7.45, oxygen to 99-100%, A1C below 5.0, CRP <1.0, Gelactin-3 <17.3%, electrolytes kept in perfect balance, and cartilage, bone, and cardiovascular state kept normalized. These markers tell us how close to "homeostasis" we have come with diet, hydration, and lifestyle.

More Resources

Brook, I. (2013). Anaerobic Infections: microbiology, diagnosis, and treatment of infections caused by anaerobic bacteria. Retrieved on July 2, 2013, from http://anaerobicinfections.blogspot.com/p/central-nervous-system-eye-and-dental.html.

Cartland, R.F. (2011). The US Dental Amalgam Debate, 2010 Meeting of the FDA Dental Products Panel. (Revised November 18, 2012)

Chartrand, M.S. (2013). Beware the Septic Keratosis Obturans: Stealth Public Health Threat (Monograph). Casa Grande, AZ: DigiCare Behavioral Research.

Chartrand, M.S. (2013). How to Raise Your Body's pH & Overcome Chronic Disease. Casa Grande, AZ: DigiCare Behavioral Research.

Griffin, R.M. (2013). Periodontal Disease and heart Health. Retrieved on July 10, 2013, from http://www.webmd.com/heart-disease/features/periodontal-disease-heart-health.

Healing Teeth Naturally (2013). Drilling & filling teeth: an unwise choice? Retrieved on July 6, from http://www.healingteethnaturally.com/drilling-filling-risks-dangers. Html.

Huggins, H. (2010, June 25). Root Canal Dangers. Retrieved on July 8, 2013 from http://www.westonprice.org/dentistry/root-canal-dangers.

Strupp, W. (2013). Cementation. Retrieved on July 2, 2013, from http://www.dentaleconomics.com/articles/print/volume-101/issue-10/personal-enrichment/.

X

Beware the Septic Keratosis Obturans:
Stealth Public Health Threat

Citation: Chartrand MS (2016) Septic Keratosis Obturans: A Stealth Public Health Threat. Otolaryngology 6: 283. doi: 10.4172/2161-119X.1000283, ISSN: 2161-119X.

Introduction: The following paper is designed to be a training monograph for general health professionals involved in cerumen management. Here is presented the septic keratosis obturans, which is commonly confused with impacted cerumen. This insidious form presents with a cerumen veneer, is rarely accompanied with complaints of pain or discomfort, and as will be shown below, can turn deadly in its final stages when one's immunology attempts to vascularize the septic mass. Since 1978 the author and associates have noted that because of a dramatic and steady increases in chronic disease in the population, that the incidence of this phenomena has likewise increased. However, the healthcare field is still responding as if it is business as usual and is a simple cerumen accumulation. The explanations given here come from a study conducted from 2002 to 2006 from a file base of more than 3000 patients in an Occupational Therapy/Hearing Health practice in Colorado [1]. This paper is intended to provide how the phenomena might be described to consumers and to the healthcare community, in general.

Impacted Earwax vs Keratosis Obturans

Often confused with ordinary earwax accumulations, insidious septic keratosis obturans appears to be increasingly common in the United States population today (Figure 1) [2]. Incidence is assumed to arise from increased prevalence in the general population of tooth/jaw sepsis, sinus infection, polypharmacy, metabolic disorders, autoimmune disorders, and chronic diseases, in general [3-6].

Healthy bodies exhibit an outer layer of tissue in the external auditory canal (EAC) called the stratum corneum, which is a thick and slowly moving keratin layer migrating outward from the umbo (center) of the ear drum at the rate of about 1mm per day. It carries with it dead skin tissues, debris, bacteria, fungi, and earwax. This is the self-cleaning mechanism of human ears or, historically, humans would be a deaf species, indeed [7,8].

When acidosis conditions set in—as a result of chronic dehydration, environmental toxicities, untreated sepsis of the jaw or teeth, upper respiratory distress, intestinal infections, or from infected implanted prostheses—the EAC keratin layer often begins to peel up from the epithelial layers below and wrap around itself over and over, trapping inside it a milieu of collected bacteria, dead skin cells, and debris over the course of months and years [9].

In many cases the keratosis obturans can become septic with an admixture of live bacteria, fungi, amoeba, and viruses : (see figure below for a typical microbial assay of a septic keratosis obturans). The author refers to this as the ear's equivalent of an ingrown toenail, where bacteria is trapped in space unreachable by one's immune system [10,11].

The growing bacteria inside the mass can inspire a cascade of proinflammatory cytokines, causing general inflammation, increased allergy, headache, and/or general discomfort throughout the body [12].

Over a period of years, the milieu grows until it has formed one, two, three, even four or more of these keratin-covered masses, leading in its final stages to vascularization of the obturans itself. Once vascularized, the body can respond in a manner not unlike an appendicitis or vascularized abscessed tooth at about year five or six of the obturans' growth.

In this chapter we are not referring to an external canal cholesteatoma, a condition that is often confused with a keratosis obturans. Nor is the author referring to the more acute and better recognized form of keratosis obturans that is characterized by pain and swelling [13], but instead a more commonly encountered form that is at once insidious and undetectable by consumers even to the point of near-total occlusion of the external ear canal.

However, upon removal, it can become painful, and usually

comes as a total surprise to the individual who, up to this point, has only been told by observing health professionals that it was "simply earwax and you might want to have it removed one of these days", without noting the potential criticality of the manifestation.

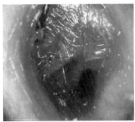

Figure 1: Septic keratosis obturans at months 3-6.

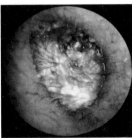

Figure 2: Septic keratosis obturans by year 5.

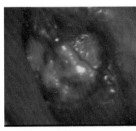

Figure 3: After Removal of the ceruminous veneer.

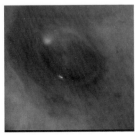

Figure 4: After Removal of 5 keratoses.

Following, is a pictorial explanation of what is too often mistaken by attending or observing health professionals as impacted earwax. In reality, however, it can be a septic keratosis obturans. When a drop in cellular pH exceeds the body's ability to maintain healthy levels—as a result of poor diet, dehydration, environmental toxicities and/or untreated sepsis of the jaw or teeth, upper respiratory distress, intestinal infections, or from infected implanted prostheses—the EAC keratin layer begins to peel up from the epithelial layers below and wraps around itself over and over, trapping inside it a milieu of collected bacteria and dead cells over the course of months and years. In many cases today it becomes dangerously septic. This is the ear's equivalent of an ingrown toenail [3,4].

Figure 1: Months 3-6. The keratin begins to insidiously peel away from the underlying skin when cellular pH (re the Krebs's cycle) of the body falls into acidosis state. The misdirected desquamated keratin continues to migrate into the space of the external canal, trapping desquamated skin cells, debris, bacteria, fungi, yeasts, pseudomonas, etc., eventually becoming septic, but remaining insulated from one's vascular system. In our observations, this formation seems to be related to the onset of diabetes type 2, tooth/jaw sepsis, egregious polypharmacy, and/or chronic upper respiratory infection. It is not a self-initiating phenomena, nor does it seem to occur as a result of just one underlying cause or contributor (Figure 3).

Figure 2: Year 5. Now, it has grown into five obturans in succession. Unresolved, they can grow into External Ear Cholesteatomas, drawing bone fragments from the mastoid bone around it, eventually hollowing out a large cavity out of the EAC. If the mass vascularizes, and septicemia reaches the blood system, lab tests will indicate an acute diverticulitis like septicemia. Immediate gentle removal is required. (Note: Often an advanced Obturans presents with a cerumen veneer, masking its serious nature to the observer. In the case at left, the individual did not complain of occlusion until a softening solution was applied)

Figure 3: After removal of the ceruminous veneer on the first obturans. When the outer debris and earwax veneer are removed by mild syringing of warm antiseptic water, revealed is the first of several keratosis- obturans. There one finds a series of membranous accumulations filled with trapped debris and growing bacteria. In the case illustrated here, there were four of these in succession, each one difficult to remove without first softening with MiraCell® Botanical Solution. They were already causing proinflammatory cytokine response elsewhere in the body and were interacting with sepsis in the teeth and jaw) (see Figure 5 for a listing of commonly found bacteria in the ear canal).

Figure 4: Complete Cascade of 5 Obturans removed. A normal eardrum is usually revealed when the final obturans is removed. An investigation of the removed objects will reveal the kinds of serious bacteria and fungi listed in a slide (Figure 5).

Note: Upon removal, a prescription by the individual's physician may be indicated for Cortisporin Ear Drops, Neomycin/Hydrocortisone or Augmentin/Hydrocortisone Ear Drops (applied 3-4 times daily for 7-10 days) followed by a two-week course of MiraCell® (or ProEar® solution by MiraCell®) botanical solution, used daily. In all cases, the cause(s) of the obturans need to found and treated (Figure 6).

Dangerous microorganisms in keratosis obturans

Bacteria/Fungi	Oto Culture	Complications
Acinetobacter lwofii	Long developing Impacted earwax	Sepsis; pneumonia; respiratory infections
Enterobacter Cloacae	Untreated injury, infection (pseudomonas)	Sepsis, pneumonia, infection
Pseudomonas aeruginosa/anaerobic	Chronic EO, EM Irritation, pH<6.5	OE, Septicemia, pneumonia
S. areus	Non-sterile earmolds, objects	Internal abscesses, carbuncles, boils
Aspergillus Favus	-pH EM, hyper-natremia, DM II (dermatitis response)	Hypersensitive pneumonitis, other systemic disease
Candida Parapsilosis	-pH EM, renal disease, thrush, DMII, gout	Candidiasis, skin Mucosal disease

[Figure 5]   DigiCare®

Introducing MiraCell's ProEAR™ Solution

17 years of reports from the field show that MiraCell's ProEar:

- Encourages keratin growth to shield the ears from bacteria and infection

- Soothes ears re adaptation of earmolds for hearing aid users

- Helps remove scar tissue, calcium plaque on eardrums

- Softens hardened earwax for easier and more natural removal

- Re-establishes pH flora of ear canal (6.50-7.35); strengthens the ear's immune system

- Use by tilting head sideways; then, pouring a generous amount into the ear canal, plugging the ear with a wad of tissue. Do the same to the other ear; let set in the ear canals for 10-15 before removing the tissue.

- Note: The above statements have not been evaluated by the FDA and must not be construed as medical diagnosis or treatment.

75

Discussion: What sets off a keratosis obturans?

As mentioned earlier, a drop in the body's cellular pH into acidosis state can cause the keratin tissue to peel up from underlying tissues in the ear canal. Today, about 120 million Americans are pre-diabetic (about 81 million) or full-blown diabetics mellitus type 2 (about 39 million, counting undiagnosed cases). Our clinical research screening protocol detects keratosis obturans in up about 25-35% in such individuals. In addition, it is often found to be co-occurring with other health conditions, such as tooth sepsis, long-term acid reflux and use of acid reflux medications, hypertension, gout, high triglycerides, IBS, and rheumatoid and osteoarthritis conditions [14-18].

Keratoses are often closely aligned to the head and neck region relative to infections in the teeth and jaw. Sepsis of the jaw appears to immunologically interact with sepsis of keratosis in the ears. Other causes that can inspire keratosis formation are:

- A serious bout of acute pneumonia, esp. fungal type, or other serious infection. Ingrown toenail and diverticulitis may also interact.
- Septic debris developing in or around implanted prostheses, such as artificial joints, shoulders, hips, knees, feet or implants in the back.
- Trauma, accident, emotional distress, or toxic exposure. "Cotton Swab Trauma" or embedment of foreign object have been implicated.
- Certain medications, especially those that suppress immune system or affect the liver, epithelium or blood vessel integrity.
- Toxic effects of tobacco, alcohol, heavy metals or drug use.

How does One Avoid Relapse?

Every case is different and are advised to consult with their physician on what may be best for them. However, here are some general guidelines to start the discussion:

- Change diet and nutrition to conform to the SIRCLE®
- Program, which helps one raise cellular pH to 7.35-7.45

- And addresses unhealed injuries and stressors that contribute negatively to one's health [19].
- Have teeth and jaw carefully examined by an oral surgeon who is intimately familiar with hidden crown/filling/ root canal problems that can harbor septicaemia [20].
- Be examined by an otologist who is knowledgeable in current trends in pseudomonas and keratosis obturans [20].
- If you have an implanted prosthesis, ask your physician about setting up a prophylactic antibiotic regimen to assure sepsis does not develop again. In most cases, Augmentin 250 mg or 500 mg taken 3 times per day for two or three days every 3 or 6 months has been advised (Rarely Ciprofloxacin) [20].
- To maintain EAC health use MiraCell on a regular basis (Figure 6) [22].

References

1. Chartrand MS (2010) Video otoscopy: A quantitative view of the relationship between external ear keratin status and success in adaptation to hearing aids. Rye, CO: DigiCare Behavioral Research.
2. Chartrand MS (2015) Incidence of keratosis obturans in an occupational therapy clinic. DigiCare Behavioral Research, Casa Grande, AZ.
3. Oral Health America (2006) A state of decay: The oral health of older Americans.
4. Rattue G (2012) Autoimmune Disease Rates Increasing. Medical News Today.
5. Thorsteinsson AL, Vestergaard P, Eiken P (2014) External auditory canal and middle ear cholesteatoma and osteonecrosis in bisphosphonate-treated osteoporosis patients: A Danish national register-based cohort study and literature review. Osteoporos Int 25: 1937-1944.
6. Roibertson DP (2015) Management of Severe Tooth Infections. BMJ.
7. Johnson A, Hawke M (1988) Non-auditory physiology of the external ear. In: Jahn AF, Santos-Sacchi J (eds.) Physiology of the ear. New York: Raven Press, pp:41-58.
8. Naiberg J, Berger G, Hawke M (1984) The pathologic features of keratosis obturans & cholesteatoma of the external auditory canal. Arch Otolaryngol 110: 690-693.
9. .Chartrand MS (2004) The importance of the keratin layer to successful fitting and treatment (Continuing Education). Livonia, Michigan: International Hearing Society.
10. Kemp RJ, Bankaitis AE (2000) Infection control for audiologists. In: Hosford-Dunn H, Roeser R, Valente M (eds.) Audiology diagnosis, treatment and practice management. Vol. III, New York: Theime Publishing Group.
11. Roland PS (2001) Chronic external otitis. Ear Nose Throat J 80: 12-16.

12. Schulte W, Bernhagen J, Bucala R (2014) Cytokines in Sepsis: Potent Immunoregulators and Potential Therapeutic Targets—An Updated View. Mediators of Inflammation 25: 1937-1944.
13. Sundstrom J, Mulligan K (2002) Neuroanatomy interactive syllabus. Ch 7: Auditory system, University of Washington.
14. Persaud RA, Hajioff D, Thevasagayam MS, Wareing MJ, Wright A (2004) Keratosis obturans and external ear canal cholesteatoma: How and why we should distinguish between these conditions. Clin Otolaryngol Allied Sci 29: 577-581.
15. Persaud RA, Hajioff D, Thevasagayam MS, Wareing MJ, Wright A (2004) Keratosis obturans and external ear canal cholesteatoma: How and why we should distinguish between these conditions. Clin Otolaryngol Allied Sci 29: 577-581.
16. Thorsteinsson AL, Vestergaard P, Eiken P (2014) External auditory canal and middle ear cholesteatoma and osteonecrosis in bisphosphonate-treated osteoporosis patients: A Danish national register-based cohort study and literature review. Osteoporos Int 25: 1937-1944.
17. Chartrand MS (2003) Video otoscopy observation and referral: The FDA red flags. The Hearing Professional, pp: 9-14.
18. Sepsis Alliance (2011) Sepsis Defined.
19. King JE (2007) Sepsis in Critical Care. Crit Care Nurs Clin North Am 19: 77-86.
20. Chartrand MS (2016) How to Get Your Health Back & Take Ownership of Your Life, Second Edition. Casa Grande, AZ: DigiCare Behavioral Research.
21. Chartrand MS (2016) Septic Dental Disorders: Unrecognized Public Health Threat. Casa Grande, AZ: DigiCare Behavioral Research.
22. Chartrand MS (2011) *Prosthetics Sepsis: Talking Paints for You and Your Doctor.* Casa Grande, AZ: DigiCare Behavioral Research.
23. Chartrand MS (2002) 960 Patient Observation Study. Orem, Utah: MiraCell, Inc.

XI

Overcoming Arthritis, Spinal Stenosis & Cartilage Degeneration

Introduction: *Many people have been led to believe that chronic conditions in human health are idiopathic (cause unknown), that one is best served by addressing symptoms (pain, primarily) over causes, and that function, once lost, is essentially irretrievable. But in the "greenhouse" environment of applied research, an entirely different picture emerges. With real people sitting in front of clinicians, it is found: 1) causal factors are no mystery when objectively examined through the prism of physical biomarkers and a thorough Case History, and 2) the body has the uncanny ability for self-repair when those causal factors are substantively addressed. Hence, the first rule of medicine when treating chronic conditions should always be to get the patient healthy. That is Job #1. Then, what's left over can be addressed through more directed care. Alas, this ideal protocol, in practice, turns out to be the rare exception, not the rule.*

Arthritis Defined

In Behavioral Medicine, arthritis is defined as *"acute or chronic inflammation of one or more joints, usually accompanied by pain and stiffness resulting from infection, heavy metal and environmental toxicity, food and food additives, gout, rheumatic fever, long-term acidosis, unhealed injury, autoimmune disease, and/or degenerative changes in the body. Pain is the body's messenger that alerts you and your immune system that something needs attention/repair. Too often, however, we 'shoot the messenger', which disengages many of the body's restorative powers, and the condition progresses to more serious disease and debilitation. This is how chronic conditions cascade into acute events."* (Chartrand, 2015)

By the foregoing we can surmise that it is indeed the rare individual who doesn't suffer from some degree or form of arthritis during their lifetime. *Osteoporosis*, or extreme loss of bone mass, is also part of the cascade as is crippling infection/injury-inspired *Rheumatoid Arthritis* (RA). Hence, arthritis is the #1 cause of disability in the United States, costing more than $220 billion dollars annually.

You'd think those high stakes would garner more than mere half measures from the healthcare community. But half measures are built into the current system, all the way from reimbursement codes to so-called "best practice standards" and, of course, business considerations. The aim here is to help consumers take a decisive step toward taking ownership of their health, not by half measures like masking pain, but by addressing forthrightly the causal factors that robbed them of their good health and function in the first place...

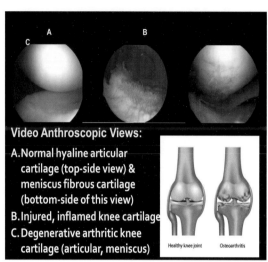

Video Anthroscopic Views:

A. Normal hyaline articular cartilage (top-side view) & meniscus fibrous cartilage (bottom-side of this view)
B. Injured, inflamed knee cartilage
C. Degenerative arthritic knee cartilage (articular, meniscus)

Healthy knee joint   Osteoarthritis

Main Types of Arthritis

There are at least 100 different classifications of arthritis. We will cover the most common ones here, with a couple of rare ones in the mix, to show range and sampling of the types currently diagnosed. More telling, however, is not the type of malady with which one suffers, but what *caused* it. Please, keep in mind that rarely is there just one stand alone cause, but often multiple and overlapping causes. Without addressing all causal factors nothing really lasting has happened. Here are some of the types of arthritis and their causes:

Osteoarthritis- Caused by long-term acidosis, nutrient deficiencies, unhealed injury, medications (for acid reflux, diabetes, hypertension, pain, etc.), weight gain, and/or sedentary lifestyle.

Rheumatoid Arthritis- Immunological and genetic predisposition, triggered by untreated infection/sepsis in another part of the body (<80% arising re hidden subclinical dental sepsis under crown, root canals).

Septic Arthritis- Open wound/surgically-induced destruction at site, dental often complicated by sepsis, as well as fungi, strep/staph, influenza, hepatitis, herpes, HIV infections. Also, causes raised blood sugar and pancreatitis, which too often is mistaken for diabetes type 2.

Gout Arthritis- Associated with loss of protease enzyme production in the stomach (re Acid Reflux Medications).

Psoriatic Arthritis- Associated with ongoing/untreated (subclinical) infection.

Lupus Arthritis- Associated with systemic lupus erythematosus (~subject to misdiagnosis).

Sjogren's Syndrome- Destruction of exocrine glands for saliva/tears; closely associated with rheumatoid arthritis, 4 mil sufferers (>90% female).

Current Practice Standards: Half Measures

Under the paradigm of addressing symptoms and leaving causal factors untouched, research reveals the following outcomes of current treatment approaches. Indeed, if one were to keep their health problem over the long-term, this is what they would do:

- Take **non-steroidal anti-inflammatories (NSAIDS)**, which draw blood, oxygen, and essential nutrients away from the site of lesion and literally turn off one's natural immunological repair system.

Non-Solutions: Long-Term Pain Killers

Opioids (Morphine, Oxycontin, Oxycodone, Percocet, Vicodin, Dilaudid, Methadone, Fentanyl, Tylenol 3, 4)

- Speeds progression of disease by destruction of autoimmunity
- As body adapts to the opium, loses effects creating side effects
- Creates new pathologies you did not have before taking them
- Cognitive & physical decline most lasting features (speeds aging)
- #1 Cause of suicides, accidental deaths in US. (twice the number of deaths from auto accidents)

Steroids (Prednisone, Cortisone, Medrol DosPak)

-Long-Term, lead to degeneration
-Safer Route: Medrol DosPak (1x every 6/12 mos)

Non-Steroidal Anti-Inflammatories (NSAIDs) (Motrin, Ibuprofin, Naprosyn, Indocin, Celebrex)

-Cause damage to liver, kidneys
-Pull blood away from lesion

Non-Constricting NSAIDs (Aspirin, Tylenol)

-Aspirin in the long-term weakens blood vessels
-"Tylenol Liver" is fast becoming a new pathology

More "Non-Solutions": Long-Term Anti-Inflammatories

- Over-use of long-term steroids has caused unbelievable harm to the public health.
- These lifesaving drugs, while quite useful in acute medicine, are only marginally useful and even dangerous to your health when used long-term for chronic conditions. Require significant judgment.
- Because the goal is often not to heal but to *manage* disease it is too often used indiscriminately, leading to greater life threatening pathologies, and an increasingly unwell population.

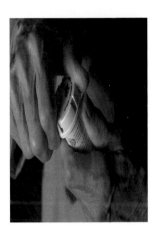

- Take **corticosteroids**, such as prednisone in high doses and for extended periods of time, letting the "party roll on" while bone mass depletes, affected cartilage fails to regenerate, and underlying causes rage on unabated.

- Take long-term **opioid pain killers**, which eventually ruin the liver and immunological functions, cause narcotic addictions, and after all is said and done, is ineffective at removing the pain it was prescribed for.

- Rely solely upon **surgery and medication** instead of making changes in one's lifestyle, diet, and health to overcome the effects of arthritis.

The Body's Amazing Ability to Self-Repair

From before birth onward, our body generates new cells—new skin, new cartilage, new bone, new muscle, and new neural and vascular tissues. We are not manikins, after all, but biologically dynamic, self-repairing organisms that continually strive to keep us up to our own unique DNA specifications. But only if we allow it do so. When we pile on too many toxic burdens and oxidative stress, the body's regenerating abilities become impaired, We age faster and experience disease. In fact, almost all chronic disease stems from that which keeps these self-repair abilities from doing their job.

Enter arthritis—-that stiffening and ossification of joints and tendons—and what has happened is usually a combination of interrupted neurology of the spine and limbs, circulatory constrictions, micronutrient deficiencies, toxic food additives, heavy metal accumulations, post-surgical or injury trauma, and yes, sedentary lifestyle (see chart to the right). In fact, if one's lifestyle remains sedentary, combined with weight gain, they may become "candidates" for things like knee and hip replacement. The question at this point will be whether or not one is willing to do what it takes to regenerate the needed new tissues, so that such surgeries are not necessary.

"Our Hero": Mitochondria, ATP & Stem Cells

From Lin et al. (2010): *"The potential to heal once incurable degenerative diseases by regenerating cells that have failed or are about to fail is now within our grasp, thanks to the emergence of regenerative medicine using adult stem cells...Their potential to differentiate into cell types found in other tissues [such as cartilage] means they can travel to the site of damage, penetrate the damaged tissue, and then regenerate this tissue by a process called transdifferentiation."*

The SIRCLE® Method begins with discovery of all contributing factors and mapping out a program for addressing each contributing factor via several core and adjunct modalities until the body is returned as closely as possible to optimal health. The principles for the therapeutic approaches are laid down in solid science and innovation. Progress is measured with ongoing Case History and Biomarker improvements.

Central to the program is lengthening of DNA and their "bookends" called telomeres, raising cellular oxygen levels as close to 100% as possible and achieving cellular pH to 7.4 (per the Kreb's cycle). Then, through stimulation of the mitochondria and its ATP production, all biomarkers begin to improve dramatically, allowing formation of more adult stem cells, which are directed to the site(s) of lesion and virtually throughout the entire body. Lost height is recovered as spinal

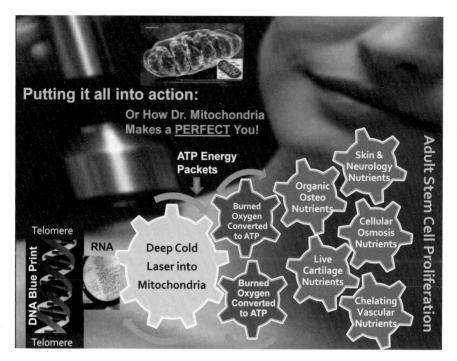

Putting it all into action:
Or How Dr. Mitochondria Makes a <u>PERFECT</u> You!

discs are repaired and expanded to their optimal size, skin becomes thicker and smoother, circulation improves all over the body, as well as re-establishment of neural tissues and bone mass. Of course, each case is different and requires different lengths of time and therapeutic attention to achieve the desired results.

Going back to the earlier stated premise, the initial goal is to achieve optimal health as quickly as possible and then see what is left over to address. Often, just getting healthy again does the trick—and getting healthy again can be a daunting task! But in cases of accumulated injuries, long standing subclinical infections requiring attention from the community healthcare team, and severe degeneration (neuropathy, diabetes, etc.), may require longer time-frames and continued targeting for the desired restorative outcomes. No half measures there. ///

Note: Other Monographs by Dr. Chartrand cover how one may benefit from adult stem cell healing with cutting edge treatment approaches. For more information: Digi-

Care Behavioral Research, 820 W. Cottonwood Lane, Suite #6, Casa Grande, AZ 85122, (520)509-6380.

Resources for Further Study

Aoshiba, K, and Nagai, A (2003). Oxidative Stress, Cell death, and Other Damage to Alveolar Epithelial Cells Induced by Cigarette Smoke. *Tobacco Induced Diseases, 1*(3):219-226)

Chakkalakal, JV, Jones, KM, Basson, MA, Brack, AS (2012). The Aged Niche Disrupts Stem Muscle Cell Quiescence. *Nature, 490*, 355-360.

Chartrand, MS (2013). *Dr. Mitochondria & You* (DVD Seminar Lecture). Casa Grande, AZ: DigiCare.

Chartrand, MS (2015). *Understanding how your own adult stem cells provide healing from injury and degeneration*, (DVD Version) Casa Grande, AZ: DigiCare.

Faloon, W. (2006). Stem Cell Therapy in a Pill? *Life Extension, December*, http://stemcells.nih.gov/staticresources/info/basics/StemCellBasics.pdf

Gnecchi, M., Zhang, Z., Ni, A, and Dzau, V (2008). Paracrine mechanisms in Adult Stem Cell Signaling and Therapy. *Circulation Research*, http://circres.ahajournals.org/content/103/11/1204.full

Jensen, FE, et al. (1994). The putative essential nutrient pyrroloquinoline quinone is a neuroprotective in a rodent model of phypoxic/ischemic brain injury. Neuroscience, 62: 2 or http://www.sciencedirect.com/science/article/pii/0306452294903751.

Lin, F. et. al. (2010). Lasers, stem cells, and COPD. Journal of Translational Medicine, 8:16, doi: 10.1186/1479-5876-8-16.

National Institutes of Health (2014). Stem Cell Information. http://stemcells.nih.gov/staticresources/info/basics/StemCellBasics.pdf

Rogerson, D., Rothenberg, R., and Marasco, W, (2007). Report: Adult Stem Cell Therapies. *Life Extension*, October, 2007.

Yu, Q., Y.S. Bai, and J. Lin, (2010). Effect of astragalus injection combined with mesenchymal stem cells transplantation for repairing the Spinal cord injury in rats. *Zhongguo Zhong Xi Yi Jie He Za Zhi*, 30(4): p. 393-7.

XII
Overcoming Neuropathy

Fibromyalgia, Peripheral & Diabetic Neuropathy, Restless Legs, Chronic Burning or Numbness, Myoclonal Jerking, etc.

Introduction: The mission of the human nervous system is to maintain homeostasis, meaning that it facilitates distribution of hormones, nutrients, oxygen, hydration, bicarbonate, and other vital resources for glandular and muscular control. The main actors in this drama are DNA, mitochondria, ATP, cytokines, neurons, axons, dendrites, synapses, myelin, astroglia, and adult stem cells. Finely tuned with incredible intelligence and self-healing properties, our nervous system is prevented from doing its needed work when interrupted by crippling surgeries and long-term use of addictive opioid, psychotropic, steroid, anti-inflammatory and neuroleptic 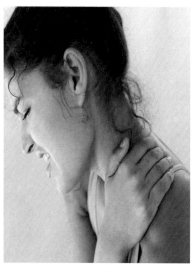 medications. Each of these only make matters worse over time, not better. To tell you how far off we are today on neuropathies in the larger scheme of things, the US consumes up to 82-84% of the world's medical grade opium with only 4% of the world population! What's worse, underlying causes are routinely ignored in favor of masking the more readily apparent symptomatic behaviors, causing those treated for neuropathic conditions in the US to rarely improve over time. Here, it is our purpose to create a greater understanding of the more than 100 recognized forms of neuropathy, and how they can be overcome. For a healthy body has a fully functioning nervous system that maintains homeostasis and wellness for an entire lifetime. (**Note:** This chapter is not exhaustive or comprehensive. For guidance in individual cases, one should seek the advice of a qualified health professional).

Neuropathy Defined

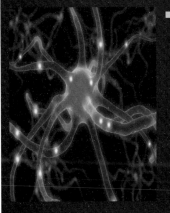

■ "Neuropathy as a chronic pathophysiological condition takes several forms: Loss of myelin (i.e., myelinated nerves) and astroglia (unmyelinated nerves); injury of nerve fiber; heavy metal and chemical neurotoxicity; oxygen/nutrient deprivation; loss of limbic control (cognitive); viral/bacterial disease and/or atrophy (as a result of disuse)."

Manifestations of Neuropathy

Neuropathies are like a lot of things in life, difficult to describe but you know it when you experience it. Sensations and discomfort and loss of function that are not visible, but they are real just the same. Some common descriptions:

- **Numbness, pain, burning, tingling**
- **Difficulty walking, unsteady gait, los of balance**
- **Muscle weakness, muscle cramps, paralysis**
- **Blurred vision, loss of vision**
- **Hearing loss, tinnitus, loudness growth abnormalities**
- **Loss of sense of taste/smell**
- **Loss of dexterity, tactile sensation**
- **Idiopathic digestive disorders**
- **Sleeplessness, loss of autonomic control, myoclonal jerking**
- **Loss (or elevation) of blood pressure, tachycardia, dizziness**
- **Loss of memory, chronic depression, cognitive dysfunction**

Afferent Nerves carry auditory, visual, tactile, olfactory, and gustatory information *toward* the brain, while ***Efferent Nerves*** transmit motor commands away *from* the brain in elaborate and dynamic pathways for responses to sensory stimuli (i.e., speech, reflexes, changes of blood pressure, heart rate, blood volume, breathing, digestion, etc.). Within various regions of the nervous system are found alternate and integrative pathways, and involuntary ***Reflex Arcs*** that facilitate immune response, protection from injury, "fight or flight" reactions, vascular variations, and systemic and digestive processes. Myoclonic jerks of the legs, for instance, are often distortions of the reflex arcs as the brain switches gears from wake-to-sleep states. Myoclonic and Occupational Overuse Syndrome (OOS) behaviors are often interactions between learned responses to stress and peripheral motor activity suggesting the need for neuromuscular retraining.

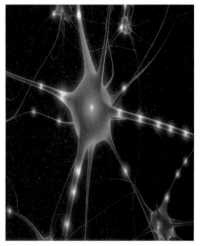

Classification

Classification of neuropathies come from several viewpoints. The first clinical descriptor delineates time-line & severity: *Acute* (immediate, debilitating), *Subacute* (recurring, less debilitating), and *Chronic* (duration of at least 3-6 months, varying levels of pain & debilitation).

Next, neuropathy is classified by *Site of Lesion*: *Cranial* (from the 12 cranial nerves of the brain), *Peripheral* (involving shoulders, hands, arms, legs, feet, hips), *Autonomic* (heart, lungs, liver, pancreas, and other involuntary organs, and spinal nerves), and *Focal* (involving one part of the body).

To learn how neuropathies develop, we will review the known primary *Causes and Contributors as follows*:

•**Diabetes mellitus type 2** tops the list of causal conditions because it is so pervasive. Most sufferers of long-term diabetes type 2 can count on experiencing neuropathy over time, particularly blindness, hearing loss, and (diabetic) peripheral neuropathy if their diabetic condition is not overcome. Amputations due to diabetes are increasing at this time.

•**Stenosis or other types of nerve compression, as well as accumulated trauma/degeneration,** arise from a lifetime of injuries and illnesses, some going back to before birth. Most are corrected without surgery, but when surgery *is* necessary, post-surgical complications may include *heterotopic ossification* of soft tissues, which can further damage or restrict the flexibility needed for connective tissues of the nervous system to function. This can cause vasculitis, blocking circulatory and immunological processes, and may also contribute to neuropathy .

•**Organic nutrition deficiencies** cause and contribute to neuropathies, especially deficiencies in the B-complex and essential minerals. A diet of microwaved, synthetically fortified, degerminated, genetically modified, refined food is a sure path to eventual neuropathies.

•**Medication & recreational drug induced neuropathies** are dramatically on the rise in the US because of over-promotion of and a seemingly bottomless pit public funding for to over-priced prescription drugs. The list of medications that can induce neuropathies is far too long to cover here. Ironically, acid reflux (GERD) medications are prominent in causing neuropathies as a result of blocking vitamin B12 and folic acid, which can cause loss of myelin insulation on the nerves (i.e., demyelination) and astroglia (the floating myelin that protects brain neurons). Long-term use of SSRI/SNRI anti-depressants, nerve deadening medications, most cardiovascular medications, and those for Alzheimer's can also contribute to development of neuropathy. As legal and illegal drug addictions rapidly rise in epidemic proportions in the US so do neuropathies and neurodegenerative conditions.

•**Heavy metal accumulations, food additives, and environmental toxins.** Lead (and a lesser degree certain other neurotoxic heavy metals) store in the bones and tissues over a lifetime and is a major contributor to neuropathies of all kinds. Even brief exposure to mercury found in commercially grown fish, fish oil supplements, and broken fluorescent bulbs and loosening dental amalgams cause varying degrees of neurological damage. Pesticides, herbicides, fluoride, chlorine, and perchlorates are all neurodegenerative, while artificial food coloring, preservatives, hormones, and artificial sweeteners that dominate the US food supply are neurotoxins especially problematic for children.

•**Acidosis** is a general biological condition inspired by microwaving food ("DNA effect"), not drinking enough water, high caffeine intake, GMO high fructose corn syrup (HFCS), stress, inflammatory disease, and unhealed injuries all contribute mightily to the development of acidosis, and in turn, can lead to neuropathy.

•**Vaccine adjuvants**, regardless of what design-biased conflict -of-interest research claim, many vaccines cause or contribute to significant developmental challenges for some infants when given too early. Neurodegenerative challenges for older adults is also a concern. Last year's flu shots caused more harm that good to the public health, according to objective reports. Caution and common sense needs to be considered in administering vaccines to those with challenged immune systems and

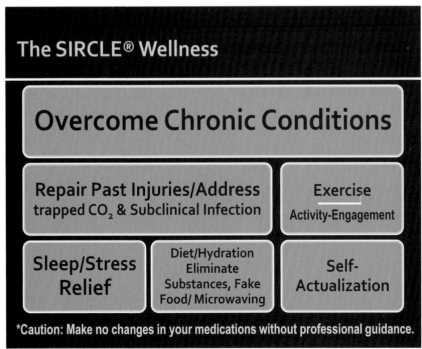

The SIRCLE® Wellness

Overcome Chronic Conditions

Repair Past Injuries/Address trapped CO_2 & Subclinical Infection

Exercise Activity-Engagement

Sleep/Stress Relief

Diet/Hydration Eliminate Substances, Fake Food/ Microwaving

Self-Actualization

*Caution: Make no changes in your medications without professional guidance.

those laden with medications and chronic conditions.

•**Infectious Disease**, including Guillain-Barre Syndrome, Shingles, Poliovirus, Rubella, Lupus, Hepatitis, HIV, Meningitis, etc. all cause or contribute to neuropathy (sensory and autonomic neuropathies).

•**Genetic Disorders** (Friedrich's Ataxia, Charcot-Marie-Tooth Disease), Hereditary Neuropathy with Liability to Pressure Palsies, etc.) also deserve listing, albeit in this researcher's opinion the vast majority of genetically inspired disease would not even occur without certain stressors, deficiencies, substances, and toxicities driving them.

As one can see from the foregoing, neuropathy appears immensely complex, yet when broken down by causal factors, we begin to understand what is needed to address it. The fact of the matter is that no drug undoes or reverses the neuropathic damage. So, the question from consumers who suffer from neuropathy complexes and syndromes is: How do we resolve my particular condition?

The answer is imbedded in first understanding the mechanisms that caused the problems and overcome them. Pain is just the messenger, the Paul Revere riding through the sleepy town of compromised immunology in our body. We should listen to him, not shoot him. He is only a symptom, not a cause.

Solutions, then, lie within reach by first recognizing the problem through mechanisms, to wit:

- *Neural Compression* (trauma, stenosis, degeneration, inflammation, tumors).
- *Demyelination* (nutrient deficiencies, medication side-effects, heavy metals, toxins, viruses).
- *Astroglia Destruction* (free radicals, toxins, food additives, drugs, deficiencies).
- *Neuronal Degeneration* (disease, acidosis, and toxicities), *Vascular Disease* (vasculitis, Factor V, hyper/hypotension, edema, hypoxia, etc.).
- *Cellular Acidosis* (dehydration, high caffeine, microwaving, over-processed diet).

These mechanisms constitute some of the challenges that need to be overcome if neuropathy is to be resolved. Although each case will be different, they will be resolved by first getting healthy and then by focusing on each relevant underlying component.

Note: Monographs by Dr. Chartrand cover hundreds of topics explaining how one may benefit from adult stem cell healing with cutting edge treatment approaches. For more information, contact: DigiCare Behavioral Research, 820 W. Cottonwood Lane, Suite #6, Casa Grande, AZ 85122, (520)509-6380.

Resources for Further Study

Chartrand, MS (2014). *What's Wrong with Microwaving?* Monograph. DigiCare Behavioral Research.

Cleveland Clinic (2014). Center for Continuing Education. http://www.clevelandclinicmeded.com/medicalpubs/ diseasemanagement/neurology/peripheral-neuropathy/.

DiabetesInControl.Com (2014). *Neuropathy*, http:// www.diabetesincontrol.com/diabetes-in-control-newsletters/neuropathy

Lee L. (1989). "Health effects of microwave radiation-microwave ovens," *Lancet*

National Institute of Neurological Disorders and Stroke. Peripheral Neuropathy Fact Sheet. http:// www.ninds.nih.gov/disorders/peripheralneuropathy/ detail_peripheralneuropathy.htm.

Retner, R. (2015). Heroin Overdose Deaths nearly Quadruple in 13 Years. Live Science, http:// www.livescience.com/50025-heroine-overdose-deaths-united-states.html

Right Diagnosis (2014). Myoclonic Jerks and Papilloedema. http://symptoms.rightdiagnosis.com/cosymptoms/ myoclonic-jerking/papilloedema-desc-sall.htm

Rust & Kissinger (2008). "BPA leaches from 'safe' products" *Journal Sentinel Online.*

Villablanca E (December 19, 2007) "Ionizing and non-ionizing radiation: Their difference and possible health consequences.

XIII

Understanding Breathing Disorders:
Allergies, Asthma, Chronic Bronchitis, COPD

Introduction: *Breathing disorders are growing at breakneck pace in the population, affecting young and old alike. Developmental delay in children ages 0-3 suffering with inhalant allergies, asthma, and otitis media with effusion (OME) is on the rise at one end of life's spectrum, while a virtual explosion is underway in acquired asthma, chronic bronchitis, and COPD in older adults. This latter condition (COPD) has risen to the number three cause of death in the US, with an expected 150,000+ deaths this year alone. Meanwhile, various research projects are finding that damaged and lost lung tissue, including pleura, alveolar I & II, clear hyaline cartilage and soft bone tissue can be repaired and replaced...without drugs... without surgery. This is groundbreaking news, but is just not reaching those who need it the most.*

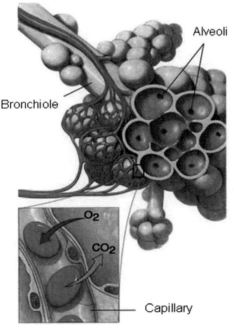

Alveoli

Bronchiole

O_2

CO_2

Capillary

First, a Review of Functional Physiology

Human lungs consist of **two large air-filled sacs within the thorax (chest cavity)** and are comprised of **epithelial cells, clear hyaline cartilage, soft bone** tissue, among other tissues. **The nose, mouth,** and **cilia** of the **trachea** filter the air we breathe and expel that which cannot be absorbed internally into the body.

The lungs **inhale oxygen (O^2)** from the trachea via **bronchial branches;** these subdivide repeatedly into smaller branches, and end in clusters of tiny air sacs called **alveoli** or **alveolar cells.** Alveolar cells give up carbon dioxide (**CO^2**) **arising from metabolic wastes of the body from the bloodstream** and take in the new O^2. O2 attaches to **hemoglobin** for wide distribution to cells throughout the body with the help of about 100,000 heart beats per day. This is the energy used by **adenosine triphosphate** (ATP), which maintains the body.

The powerful **diaphragm** muscles beneath the lungs enable the lungs to expand to take air in and contract to push air outward approximately 20,000 times each day. To assure no friction occurs in the expansion and contraction cavity, there is a thin, wet layer of cells called the **pleura**, which slides against the pleural lining on the inside of the thorax.

Dead cells, mucus, and infection are absorbed by **macrophage cells** into the **vascular** (blood) and **lymphatic systems**, or we would all be

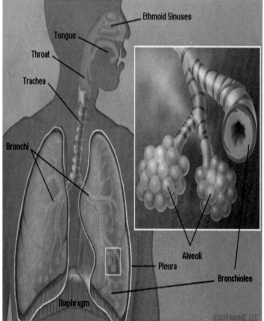

Ethmoid Sinuses
Tongue
Throat
Trachea
Bronchi
Alveoli
Pleura
Bronchioles
Diaphragm

©2003 WebMD, LLC

Cascade for Breathing Disorders

CHILDHOOD	ALLERGIES	Asthma	Chronic Bronchitis	COPD
DEVELOPMENTAL STRESSORS: -Premature birth -Low birth weight -Lead in water/food/air -Too early vaccines -Mother's smoking -Second-hand smoke -Ear infections [OME] -Bronchitis/Pneumonia -Childhood Asthma* (* less than 20% diagnosed)	Overuse of antibiotics & steroids increase sensitivities to environmental and food toxins. Celiac disease, "hay fever", severe headache, & compromised immunology lead to worsened health issues (seemingly unrelated to each other)	Each case different: many began with [childhood] respiratory stressors. Others develop from spinal stenosis, tooth & jaw sepsis, acidosis and/or long-term use of medications	In tandem with other degenerative states (i.e., acidosis, atherosclerosis, spinal stenosis, nutritional deficiencies, antibiotic overuse, polypharmacy) ---many of these will cascade into full-blown COPD over the long-term	Lifestyle stress, past infections, environmental hazards, and/or long-term meds destroy bronchiole, alveolar, callogen & pleural cells; This year more than 150,000 Americans will die from COPD. <35% never smoked.

The good news is that nearly ALL cases of breathing disorders can be improved dramatically when underlying causes & over-all health are addressed , coupled with therapeutic regeneration of

coughing virtually round the clock. In their normal, healthy state lung tissues **regenerate in cycles of 7-21 days**. Cartilage and bone cells replenish over several months, depending on one's level of physical activity. When these cells are under constant attack by airborne particulates, toxins, infection, smoke, and/or certain medications (steroids, antihistamine, NSAIDs), timely regeneration is delayed or stopped entirely. The degree to which such degeneration occurs can often be aligned with the diagnoses of **acquired asthma, chronic bronchitis, emphysema, COPD**.

Lung functions are intricately connected to **limbic control** (emotion/thought) and the **immune system** (external & internal threats/triggers). These relationships affect stress reactions and cardiovascular functions, including blood pressure.

Most cases of upper and lower respiratory abnormalities began at birth from stressors present at the time of birth (mother's health state, egregious medications, smoking, withdrawal, etc.). A diet devoid of needed organic micronutrients plus overuse of antibiotics to treat allergy-related OME and repeated bouts of chronic bronchitis, tonsillitis, and/or pneumonia combine to slow a child's cartilaginous, neurological, and cognitive development.

Many of these, with added years of lifestyle and workplace stressors carry over into older adulthood, making those with earlier stressors to comprise the largest segment of today's serious breathing disorder cases.

Recent research demonstrates that regeneration of **fully functioning respiratory** cells are attainable via generation of adult stem cells. However, the chasm between one's current state and the state where their lungs *can* regenerate is usually difficult to cross due to **aggressive symptomatic treatment** and the disregard **for addressing underlying causes.** Addressing underlying and contributing factors (i.e., biomarkers), as well as building up the health of the entire body is what the **SIRCLE® Method** is all about.

We refer readers to other monographs that discuss how damaged and missing tissues can be grown back under the right circumstances and treatment protocols. Hence, the needed advanced organic nutritive components to encourage adult stem cell growth and technology that can dramatically increase ATP repair is available for the asking, today!

Note: Monographs by the author cover how one may benefit from adult stem cell healing with cutting edge therapeutic approaches. For more information, contact: DigiCare Behavioral Research, 820 W. Cottonwood Lane, Suite #6, Casa Grande, AZ 85122, (520)509-6380.

For Further Study

Aoshiba, K, and Nagai, A (2003). Oxidative Stress, Cell death, and Other Damage to Alveolar Epithelial Cells Induced by Cigarette Smoke. *Tobacco Induced Diseases, 1*The Aged Niche Disrupts Stem Muscle Cell Quiescence. *Nature, 490,* 355-360.

Chartrand, MS (2013). *Dr. Mitochondria & You* (DVD Lecture). Casa Grande, AZ: DigiCare.

Chartrand, MS (2015). *Understanding how your own adult stem cells provide healing from injury and degeneration,* (DVD Version) Casa Grande, AZ: DigiCare.

Dean, C., Bingle, C., and Hind, M. (2013). Delivering and phenotyping mouse models for the respiratory community. *Clin Sci (London), November; 125*(10):495-500.

Faloon, W. (2006). Stem Cell Therapy in a Pill? *Life Extension, December,* http://stemcells.nih.gov/static resources/info/basics/StemCellBasics.pdf

Gray, B (2012). Study gives first evidence that human lungs can regrow. *HealthDay,* July, 2012.

Healthline News, (2015). Asthma and Allergies on the Rise in the US. At http://www.healthline.com/health-news/children-allergies-and-asthma-on-the-rise-110813.

Penn Medicine (2015). Limber Lungs: One Type of Airway Cell Can Regenerate Another Lung Cell Type. At http://www.uphs.upenn,edu/news/news_release/2015/04/epstein. (3):219-226)

Chakkalakal, JV, Jones, KM, Basson, MA, Brack, AS (2012). The Aged Niche Disrupts Stem Muscle Cell Quiescence. *Nature, 490,* 355-360.

Chartrand, MS (2013). *Dr. Mitochondria & You* (DVD Lecture). Casa Grande, AZ: DigiCare.

Chartrand, MS (2015). *Understanding how your own adult stem cells provide healing from injury and degeneration,* (DVD Version) Casa Grande, AZ: DigiCare.

Dean, C., Bingle, C., and Hind, M. (2013). Delivering and phenotyping mouse models for the respiratory community. *Clin Sci (London), November;* *125*(10):495-500.

Faloon, W. (2006). Stem Cell Therapy in a Pill? *Life Extension, December,* http://stemcells.nih.gov/staticresources/info/basics/StemCellBasics.pdf

Gray, B (2012). Study gives first evidence that human lungs can regrow. *HealthDay,* July, 2012.

Healthline News, (2015). Asthma and Allergies on the Rise in the US. At http://www.healthline.com/health-news/children-allergies-and-asthma-on-the-rise-110813.

Penn Medicine (2015). Limber Lungs: One Type of Airway Cell Can Regenerate Another Lung Cell Type. At http://www.uphs.upenn,edu/news/news_release/2015/04/epstein.

XIV

Overcoming

Diabetes Mellitus & Borderline Diabetes

As a Behavioral Medicine Consultant I've long been concerned about the skyrocketing rates of diabetes and pre-diabetes in the United States, growing 13 times per capita since 1970. Here we will address the reasons this is happening and how these trends may be reversed. Indeed, more than 90% of cases *can* be reversed, if one is willing to take charge and actually make the changes required to make it happen.

As will be explained in greater detail later, reversal of diabetic behaviors would require, at the least, a marked change

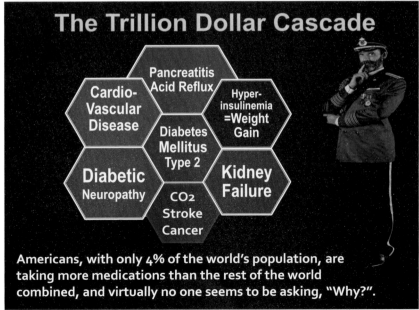

The Trillion Dollar Cascade

Pancreatitis Acid Reflux

Cardio-Vascular Disease

Hyper-insulinemia =Weight Gain

Diabetes Mellitus Type 2

Diabetic Neuropathy

Kidney Failure

CO_2 Stroke Cancer

Americans, with only 4% of the world's population, are taking more medications than the rest of the world combined, and virtually no one seems to be asking, "Why?".

of diet (comprising at least 50% fresh fruits/vegetables), refraining from eating GMO high fructose corn syrup, stopping all microwaving of foods, and avoiding where possible other offenders that dominate the American food supply (Aspartame, MSG, Bromides, Canola Oil, etc.). Other factors that are also important are to resolve sepsis and subclinical infections in the body (teeth, ears, around prosthetic joints), nonsurgical repair of past injuries, and oral chelation of heavy metals and arterial plaques.

Getting to root causes of conditions like high blood pressure, elevated triglycerides, and other biomarkers *without prescription drugs* is also necessary, for most of the associated medications actually *cause* or exacerbate diabetes and weight gain! Assuring appropriate exercise and weight loss (if needed) are part of that which will help one overcome developing diabetes.

The over-arching biomarkers that have more to do with the ability to restore normal metabolic processes is in achieving a cellular pH 7.45 (via the Kreb's Cycle) and blood oxygen at 99% (per the glycolysis cycle). At the least, getting one's cellular pH to 7.45 and A1CHg score (a measure of hemoglobin)

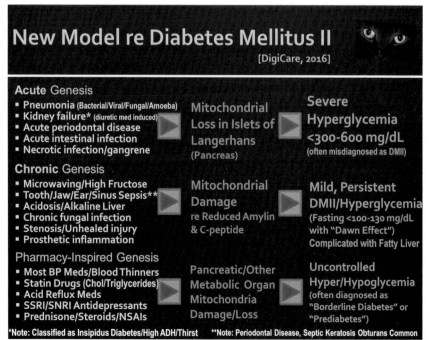

New Model re Diabetes Mellitus II
[DigiCare, 2016]

Acute Genesis
- Pneumonia (Bacterial/Viral/Fungal/Amoeba)
- Kidney failure* (diuretic med induced)
- Acute periodontal disease
- Acute intestinal infection
- Necrotic infection/gangrene

Mitochondrial Loss in Islets of Langerhans (Pancreas)

Severe Hyperglycemia <300-600 mg/dL
(often misdiagnosed as DMII)

Chronic Genesis
- Microwaving/High Fructose
- Tooth/Jaw/Ear/Sinus Sepsis**
- Acidosis/Alkaline Liver
- Chronic fungal infection
- Stenosis/Unhealed injury
- Prosthetic inflammation

Mitochondrial Damage re Reduced Amylin & C-peptide

Mild, Persistent DMII/Hyperglycemia (Fasting <100-130 mg/dL with "Dawn Effect") Complicated with Fatty Liver

Pharmacy-Inspired Genesis
- Most BP Meds/Blood Thinners
- Statin Drugs (Chol/Triglycerides)
- Acid Reflux Meds
- SSRI/SNRI Antidepressants
- Prednisone/Steroids/NSAIs

Pancreatic/Other Metabolic Organ Mitochondria Damage/Loss

Uncontrolled Hyper/Hypoglycemia (often diagnosed as "Borderline Diabetes" or "Prediabetes")

*Note: Classified as Insipidus Diabetes/High ADH/Thirst   **Note: Periodontal Disease, Septic Keratosis Obturans Common below 6.0 can be a daunting task! See the chart "Cellular pH vs Chronic Disease" to the left to get an idea of the relationship between human disease and cellular pH—these are strong correlations! Cellular pH *cannot* easily be determined from blood pH, nor from urine, saliva, or hair, contrary to some opinions.

To-date, only Video Otoscopy Biomarker Assessment, as developed by the author and colleagues over nearly four decades of research and development, has shown to be a reliable *and* low cost way to assess one's long-term cellular pH level (aka acid-alkaline balance per the Kreb's cycle). Biopsy, needless to say, is exorbitant in cost and requires one to actually be present at the lab at the time of the assay to be accurate.

From the above model titled *"The Diabetes Cascade"*, one can see the primary chronic conditions that develop concurrently with and/or *because of* diabetes. For instance, one needs to keep in mind that when insulin is in the bloodstream for more than a short period of time two to three times a day, it nearly always causes one to take on more body fat and muscles begin resisting oxygen, insulin, and glucose simultaneously. This brings muscle wasting!

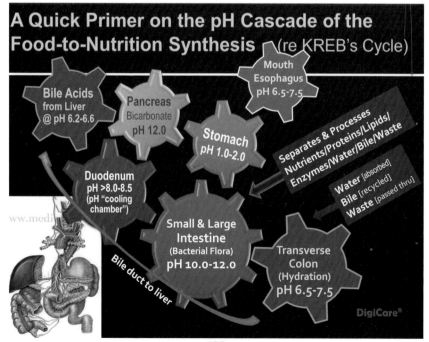

A Quick Primer on the pH Cascade of the Food-to-Nutrition Synthesis (re KREB's Cycle)

Mouth Esophagus
pH 6.5-7.5

Bile Acids from Liver @ pH 6.2-6.6

Pancreas Bicarbonate pH 12.0

Stomach pH 1.0-2.0

Separates & Processes Nutrients/Proteins/Lipids/ Enzymes/Water/Bile/Waste

Water [absorbed]
Bile [recycled]
Waste [passed thru]

Duodenum pH >8.0-8.5 (pH "cooling chamber")

Small & Large Intestine (Bacterial Flora) pH 10.0-12.0

Transverse Colon (Hydration) pH 6.5-7.5

Bile duct to liver

DigiCare®

Common trends that are driving the growing pandemic of diabetes, obesity, CVD, cancer, and related chronic diseases in the US are:

●A genetically modified, irradiated, synthetically fortified, degerminated, over-processed, micronutrient empty, microwaved diet!

●A five-fold per capita increase in intake of caffeine, high fructose in particular, and harmful artificial sweeteners since 1980. There are NO safe artificial sweeteners!

●Sedentary lifestyle in the general population; Phys Ed removed from the public schools in the US with disastrous results!

●As health declines (i.e., acid reflux, inflammatory disease, hypertension, etc.) most medications used for *these* conditions can *also lead to development of diabetes*!

●Unresolved infections and unhealed injuries that have accumulated and increasingly limit one's function and health over time.

●Increased levels of heavy metal & environmental toxicities that weaken mitochondrial DNA, and introduce unneeded metabolic and immunological stressors.

As examples of some of the little understood (septic) infections that can spike blood sugar and appear to be diabetic when such is not the case, or may cause one who *is* diabetic to have uncontrollable blood sugar, the author refers readers to the graphic on the next page titled *"Tooth Sepsis, Neuropathies, Ingrown Toenails & Prosthetic Joint Infections"* . These not only cause blood sugar to go out of control, but also cause *inflammation,* which contributes to other problems from depression (cortical inflammation), cardiac event (arrhythmias, infarct), and/or stroke (including TIAs). Timely treatment of same is of utmost importance!

Likewise, another threat that requires video otoscopy for detection: *Keratosis Obturans of the External Ear Canal.* Keratosis predominate more and more in the diabetic and pre-diabetic population today. Rarely are such recognized by health professionals, instead assuming impacted earwax im-paction—but a culture of the bacteria trapped inside will show otherwise!

Meanwhile, entrenched cottage industries have been built around each segment of these diseases, from extra hospital emergency room and clinic visits, a plethora of unnecessary tests, and overprescribed pharmaceuticals to elaborate mar-keting campaigns, elaborate investment schemes, and mil-lions of jobs...these, in turn, unwittingly disincentivizes the "business" of healthcare from applying the findings of re-search that show how these symptomatic syndromes may be resolved by changes in the food supply and better health hab-its.

It is also critical to note that despite notions to the contra-ry, insulin is a *crisis* hormone and not meant to be secreted 24/7 in the bloodstream as one would be led to believe by the way diabetes is treated today in the US. The current approach has caused unfathomable harm to our population! Every cause of elevated blood sugar needs to be addressed if one hopes to resolve diabetes. To summarize, here is a partial list-ing of crucial factors to address if one truly wishes to over-come their diabetes:

- Refrain from microwaving your food, even for warming. In-sist the restaurants and other places you at which you eat also avoid microwaving your food.

- Avoid GMO High Fructose Corn Syrup (HFCS) like the plague—check the labels—learn to use "Stevia in the Raw" with a bit of organic cane sugar to moderate taste.

- Avoid high caffeine drinks—yes, high caffeine raises blood sugar as well as depletes adrenals and weakens severely immunology! Diet drinks are deadly!

- Drink adequate filtered water—generally a glass of water every other hour during waking hours, the size of the glass dependent on one's body weight and activity level.

- Eat at least 50% of your diet in fresh fruits & vegetables, whole grains, with as little processed food as possible

- Have teeth checked carefully for sepsis under crowns and under fillings, floss daily, and take immaculate care of your teeth. Sepsis can be impossible to find in x-ray!

- Chelate lead and other heavy metal accumulations from the body with CardioFlow (other attenuated oral chelate); nearly everyone today has significant lead stored in their bones, which generally does not show up in blood tests.

- Resolve any other subclinical infections (such as inflammation around artificial knees, hips, back, etc.)—these are notorious for causing DMII.

- Check all prescription medications that contribute to or exacerbating—most hypertension/edema meds, statins, SSRI/SNRI anti-depressants, nerve blocks, pain meds, and acid reflux meds contribute mightily to diabetes. Resolve the underlying cause of the conditions causing these conditions so as not to need to take these and other side-effect laden medications in the long term.

- Repair any unhealed injuries in your body with an advanced Deep Cold Laser/Adult Stem Cell —old whiplashes, stenosis, spondylitis in neck & shoulders, neuropathy developing in the legs, or a variety of other injury caused conditions that occur over a lifetime.

- Resolve acid reflux and other digestive issues so that acid reflux medications are no longer needed—these are arguably among the most harmful medications when used in the long term, causing bone loss, metabolic imbalances, and other serious disease.

Mild pancreatitis (inflamed pancreas), along with troubling digestive conditions arising therefrom (acid reflux, celiac disease, Crohn's, IBS, to name but a few), can also mimic many of the symptoms of diabetes mellitus. Bone loss (osteoarthritis, osteopenia, osteoporosis) results from not enough bicarbonate being secreted by an inflamed pancreas, and cancer, which loves an acid environment, arise in too many cases.

Look at the chart on Targets below. These are the targets that represent an optimally healthy body, one where you "own your health" and are free of drugs and illness. *Reach these targets & watch your life get better as you get healthier and happier by the day!*

SIRCLE®: *Naturally* Achieved Targets

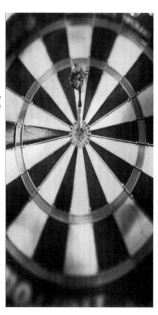

- Cellular pH 7.35-7.45

- Oxygen 98-100% @55-65 bpm

- Resting Blood Pressure: 110-135/65-80 mmHg (differs male vs female)

- Fasting blood sugar consistently <70-85 mg/dL or 3.5-5.5 mmol/L

- HgA1C score: 4.5-5.5%

- HDL: 50-80 mg/dL; LDL: 100 -140 mg/dL; triglycerides: <140 mg/dL

Note: Monographs by Dr. Chartrand cover hundreds of topics explaining how one may benefit from adult stem cell healing with cutting edge treatment approaches. For more information, contact: DigiCare Behavioral Research, 820 W. Cottonwood Lane, Suite #6, Casa Grande, AZ 85122, (520)509-6380.

XV

Adverse Effects of Hearing Loss on Mental & Physical Health

Author's Note: This contribution to the literature is designed as a consumer education primer to increase awareness among consumers and their primary medical professionals about the deleterious health effects of untreated hearing loss and tinnitus.

Introduction: Hearing Loss

More than 40 million Americans suffer from various degrees of hearing loss. The clear majority of these also have associated tinnitus annoyance. There are more people under the age of 60 with hearing los than there are over the age of 60, albeit the per capita concentration of hearing loss is much higher in the over 65 age group.

Hence, incidence of hearing loss is steadily growing in the general population, and, at least in the United States, is increasing into the younger ages. Hearing loss occurs because of congenital stressors, developmental delays, early ear infections, acoustic trauma, food additives, tooth/jaw sepsis migrating to the EAC, polypharmacy and environmental toxicity, and as a consequence of chronic diseases, such as diabetes, neuropathy, osteoarthritis, and cardiovascular disease.[1]

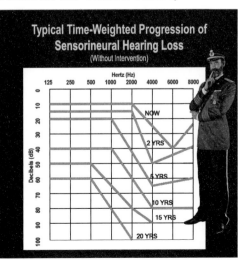

Typical Time-Weighted Progression of Sensorineural Hearing Loss
(Without Intervention)

What's even less known to many is that when hearing loss is corrected, remarkable improvements in cognitive and health performance are likewise noted. Children perform better in school, possess more in control of emotions, sleep better, and develop faster.[2] Those of working age are more productive, make higher wages, and are promoted more often.[3] Older adults with optimal hearing are healthier, take far fewer medications, need fewer medical services, and retain memory and mental acuity.[4]

This paper reviews recent research findings in hearing loss and tinnitus effects on general health, cognition, and quality of life. For those in denial, which just happens to be the biggest deterrent for seeking hearing help,[5] the cat's out of the bag: Better hearing means a better you in every way!

Tinnitus, Sensorineural Hearing Loss, and 4,000 Hz

Of all species of living creatures, humans hear the high pitch tone of 4000 Hz best of all. Hence, when humans lose that region of frequencies of 3,000-4,000 Hz, a number of important health anomalies appear: the heart's pericardial sac becomes stressed, blood pressure elevates, stress levels rise, and sleep disorders occur.[6] Notice, in figure 1 (above) that the most notable change as hearing acuity decreases over time is the notch at 4KHz. This region is also associated with loss of

Psychosocial Barriers from Uncorrected Hearing Loss

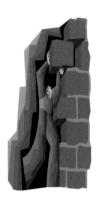

- Repetition, missed subtext
- Loud voices, lack of intimate communication
- Aversive body language, facial expressions
- Inattention (feigned or real)
- Embarrassment, defensiveness ("Fear of being found out", "deaf nod")
- Distrust, unexplainable depression & anxiety
- Isolation, loneliness, social invisibility

Question: Who on earth would ever associate these problems with lack of hearing acuity? Caveat: Recruitment, cochlear distortions, and reduced loudness discomfort levels are the hidden booby traps of sensorineural hearing loss. DigiCare®

consonantal clarity in speech and speech-in-noise ability, spatial function, chronic depression, anxiety, learning, short-term memory and cognitive health. Hearing loss of this type affects men at least 2.8:1 over women.[7]

For those with long-term tinnitus associated with their hearing loss, the 3000-4000Hz region is often described as a "high pitch ring" and is heard by millions of hearing impaired individuals in the U.S. Invariably, this means the cochlear hair cell degeneration of the frequencies around 3,000-4000 Hz (and above) are causing a sympathetic tone not unlike the "phantom limb effect" of an amputation. This researcher has described tinnitus in this range as "the search party sent in search of the missing hearing; once found—through amplification and/or medical treatment--the search party is called off and the intensity of the sound decreases and annoyance is reduced".[8]

It just happens that this pitch is also near or at the sinus node tone of the heart. This explains the strong correlation between long-standing sensorineural hearing loss and hypertension, as well as the number of medications being prescribed to control the hypertension.[9]

Such artifacts are usually caused by an advancing high frequency hearing loss that needs attention, causing a decrease in understanding the consonant sounds of speech, speech defects, and most especially difficulty understanding speech in noise. These set up hearing loss sufferers for psychological and psychosocial challenges to their quality of life and in social relationships.[10] Consequently, it is vital that the correction of high frequency loss through amplification be considered important for your lifestyle, social, occupational, and communicative well-being.

Recent research shows that hearing loss sufferers...

Utilize medical services five times as much as normal hearing individuals.[11]

Suffer cardiovascular events and hypertension from two to three times as often as their normal hearing counterparts.[12, 13]

<92% of older adults that were diagnosed with Alzheimer's disease also had uncorrected hearing loss.[14]

Mild hearing loss increases Alzheimer's risk 2x, moderate hearing loss 3x, and severe loss 5x.[15]

Uncorrected hearing loss is associated with brain shrinkage of certain areas of the brain critical for memory and other cognitive functions.[16]

Other significant health/hearing loss associations

Brandeis University Study (2006) in a PETT scan/ glucose study on short-term memory found that hearing loss causes the brain of hearing impaired individuals to burn so much glucose that simple tasks like responding in conversation or in classrooms become challenging.[17]

National Council on Aging Study (2013) found that uncorrected hearing loss "significantly and negatively impacted quality of life for older adults."[18]

Better Hearing Institute Study (2012) found that working age hearing loss sufferers make an average of $12,000 less in annual wages than workers with normal hearing in the United States.[19]

Brandeis University Study (2012) on tinnitus found that serious tinnitus can burn as much brain glucose during

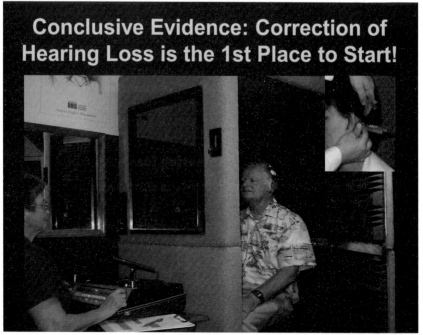

Conclusive Evidence: Correction of Hearing Loss is the 1st Place to Start!

sleep as reading a book while awake, causing chronic fatigue syndrome-like symptoms.[20]

Consumer Guidelines for Assessment, Remediation & Treatment

Build your personal case history by documenting past ear infections, exposure to loud noise (occupational and recreational), balance issues, and tinnitus.

Have your hearing tested annually, starting with a baseline audiogram and note than when it reaches the type of audiogram noted at year 2 to 5 and ask for a trial of amplification to see if it improves your communication, health, and overall well-being.

If your hearing loss is quite significant (like year 10 above), inquire about assistive technologies & coping strategies that can assist in critical and large area listening situations.

If you develop ringing of the ears (tinnitus), inquire about available solutions, such as special digital hearing aid programming, dietary and medication changes, and necessary ear protection to try to make the tinnitus softer and less bothersome.

Do not accept a mental health diagnoses for Alzheimer's/dementia as conclusive without addressing hearing loss first. No mental health assessment in older adults is valid without first identifying and resolving the auditory component.

Locate a reputable hearing health clinic that knows you and respects your need to maintain your best hearing health and stick with them!

References

1. Hearing Link (2017). What is sensorineural hearing loss? Found at https://www.hearinglink.org/your-hearing/types-causes-of-hearing-loss/what-is-sensorineural-hearing-loss/.

2. CDC (2017). Hearing Loss in Children: Treatment and Intervention. https://www.cdc.gov/ncbddd/hearingloss/treatment.html.

3. Better Hearing Institute (2017). Address Hearing Loss in the Workplace and Reap the Rewards. http://www.betterhearing.org/news/address-hearing-loss-workplace-and-reap-rewards.

4. Johns Hopkins Medicine (2017). Hidden Risks of Hearing Loss. http://

www.hopkinsmedicine.org/health/healthy_aging/.

5. Kochkin, S. (2007). MarkeTrak VII: Obstacles to adult non-user adoption of hearing aids. *Better Hearing Institute.* http://www.betterhearing.org/sites/default/files/hearingpedia-resources/M7_Barriers_to_hearing_aid_usage.pdf.

6. Chartrand, M.S. (2004). Tinnitus Retraining Therapy and Concepts of Amplification. Http://ihsinfo.org/IhsV2/hearing professional/2003/020_March-pril/030_Tinnitus_Retraining.cfm .,

7. Staab, W. (1990). Hearing in the Elderly, Part II. *Audecibel, Spring,1990.* pp. 16-22.

8. Chartrand, MS (2017). *Tinnitus & Amplification.* DigiCare Behavioral Research, CE Seminar.

9. Mondelli, MF & Lopez, AC (2009). Relation Between Arterial Hypertension and Hearing Loss. *International Archives of Otolaryngology, 13*; No. 1, Jan/Mar.

10. Chartrand, M.S. (2007). An Exploration of Psychological and Physiological Causes of Failure to Fit. http://www.audiologyonline.com/articles/exploration-psychological-physiological-causes-for-940.

11. Kochkin, S. (2013). The Impact of treated hearing loss on quality of life. *Better Hearing Institute,* http://www.betterhearing.org/aural_education_and_counseling/articles_tip_sheets_and_guides/hearing_loss_treatment /quality_of_life_detail.cfm.

12. Chartrand, M.S. (1999). *Hearing Instrument Counseling: Practical Applications in Counseling the Hearing Impaired, 2nd edition.* Livonia, MI: Intl Institute Hrg Instr Studies.

13. Science Daily (2017). Hearing Impairment News. https://www.sciencedaily.com/news/mind_brain/hearing_loss/

14. Chartrand, MS (2005). Undiagnosed Pre-Existing Hearing Loss in Alzheimer's Disease Patients? AudiologyOnline, http://www.audiologyonline.com/articles/undiagnosed-pre-existing-hearing-loss-1009.

15. Johns Hopkins Medicine (2011). Hearing Loss and Dementia Linked in Study. http://www.hopkinsmedicine.org/news/media/releases/hearing_loss_and_dementia_linked_in_study

16. Johns Hopkins Medicine (2014). Hearing Loss Linked to Accelerated Brain Tissue Loss. http://www.hopkinsmedicine.org/news/media/releases/hearing_loss_linked_to_accelerated_brain_tissue_loss

17. Science Daily (2005). Brandeis Study: Poor Hearing May Cause Poor Memory. https://www.sciencedaily.com/releases/2005/09/050901071906.htm

18. McCarthy, P., and Roeser, R. (2013). Hearing Loss Counseling (Auditory Rehabilitation). http://www.betterhearing.org/hearing_loss_treatment/hearing_loss_counseling/index.cfm.

19. Better Hearing Institute (2017). Address Hearing Loss in the Workplace and Reap the Rewards. http://www.betterhearing.org/news/address-hearing-loss-workplace-and-reap-rewards.

20. Vestibular Disorders Association (2017). Tinnitus: Ringing of the Ears, An Overview. https://vestibular.org/sites/default/files/page_files/Tinnitus%20Ringing%20in%

XVI

Keep Your Memory for Life:

A Primer on How to Avoid & Overcome Alzheimer's

Human cognition is one's awareness and consciousness of self, others, and environs around them. Cognition involves logic, knowledge, skills, critical thinking, and lifelong retention of same. Some of one's cognition is derived from countless past generations who developed various traits and reactions for survival.

These are stored in several parts of the brain, including the amygdala, seat of fight or flight responses. The lion's share of *acquired* cognition, however, is learned during one's own lifetime. Re*cognition* (or memory) is the implementation of intuitive and acquired knowledge and experience.

Amazingly, due to the plasticity of the brain, these abilities can be retained easily past 100 years of age, but *only if* diet,

The New Open Systems Model for
MEMORY LOSS IN OLDER ADULTS

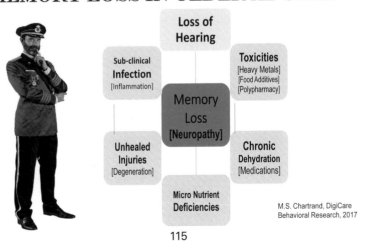

Loss of Hearing

Sub-clinical Infection [Inflammation]

Toxicities [Heavy Metals] [Food Additives] [Polypharmacy]

Memory Loss [Neuropathy]

Unhealed Injuries [Degeneration]

Chronic Dehydration [Medications]

Micro Nutrient Deficiencies

M.S. Chartrand, DigiCare Behavioral Research, 2017

hydration, sleep, exercise, refraining from toxins (tobacco, alcohol, drugs, over-medication, heavy metals, food additives, such as GMO high fructose corn syrup, GMO 24-chromosome wheat, aspartame, high caffeine, etc. Many prescription medications, for instance, can cause a cascade of *proinflammatory cytokines and* chronic semi-dehydration dehydration that make the soft tissues of the brain shrink over time, bringing dementias.

Uncorrected hearing loss is also associated with memory loss, shrinking brain tissue, raised blood pressure, and over-diagnosis of Alzheimer's. From almost four decades of research there is emerging evidence that addressing underlying causes of dementia is indeed possible to regain memory and cognition. More importantly, memory loss can be prevented in the first place. Uncorrected hearing loss also looks and quacks a lot like Alzheimer's even to the most sophisticated mental health professional (see chart below).

Symptomatic comparison: AD & HL

Late Onset Alzheimer's	Untreated Hearing Loss
Depression, anxiety, disorientation	Depression, anxiety, social isolation
Reduced language comprehension	Reduced speech discrimination
Impaired memory (esp. short-term)	Reduced cognitive input into memory
Inappropriate psychosocial responses	Inappropriate psychosocial responses
Loss of recognition (agnosia)	Reduced mental scores (cognitive dysfunction)
Denial, defensiveness, negativity	Denial, defensiveness, negativity
Distrust, suspicion of other's motives	Distrust, paranoia (e.g., belief that others are talking about them) Chartrand, 1991

The Case of the Shrinking Brain

John, aged 82 and a recent widower, had just come from his family doctor with a prescription for Aricept and Namenda, two controversial drugs for Alzheimer's, even though John showed no signs of dementia—they were prescribed "just to be sure". During the year after taking these and other medications, John went downhill in the proverbial handbasket. MRIs revealed a shrinking brain, and he finally started exhibiting the traits of one suffering from Alzheimer's. Going from walking without effort to a cane to walking frame and eventually a wheelchair, and now 11 prescription medications later, John was leading the lifestyle of a hermit; microwaved TV dinners became his total diet and he rarely drank any water.

One evening, his daughter Mary took him to a consumer seminar on how to lower blood pressure without drugs. They were surprised to find that by addressing underlying causes of hypertension—i.e., chronic dehydration, sedentary lifestyle, nutritional deficiencies, certain food additives, and acid-promoting diet—that he could indeed get his blood pressure back to normal without the three medications he was taking. His daughter also learned that the 80 mg. of statin drug that he was taking for cholesterol was also recognized for bringing on memory and motor loss in older adults. Time to change, they decided. A recent Oxford study showed eating an apple a day really *can* lower cholesterol as well as other changes in diet. With the help of a wellness-oriented physician, John was able to wean off of his dementia drugs, the statin drug, and as his blood pressure started coming down, as well.

He began eating a diet high in fresh fruits and vegetables, and fresh cooked foods; no more microwaving, not even for warming.

He increased his water intake to six glasses of water a day. He slept better, started waking up with more energy and a yearning to do things. The wheelchair, the walker, the cane *all* went into storage as he resumed his morning walks to the post office. He had his teeth fixed and started taking better care of them.

Another seminar with his daughter, this time about the John's Hopkins study that revealed the strong association between uncorrected hearing loss and loss of memory and cognition—a more recent Johns Hopkins study even found that the brains of those with uncorrected hearing loss suffer more brain shrinkage than their normal hearing counterparts.

His daughter took him in for a hearing test and from there he came home with two tiny open-ear digital hearing aids, hearing the birds chirping in the trees for the first time in years! He resumed attending church and the Lion's Club again, to the cheers of longtime friends.

He yearned to be independent, and not have to rely on others taking him everywhere. But his driver's license, check-writing powers, and about all legal authority had been taken away from him from the moment his doctor placed him on the dementia drugs. Now he had to prove he was mentally and physically fit. He studied until he "had it all down" and passed the driver's exam.

Now, 85 years young, John drove his once mothballed SUV to the post office like a one-man parade, waving at everyone he saw. What a sight to see. The hero returns to his former self, glad to be back with those he loves. Indeed, against all odds, the man with the [formerly] shrunken brain is back!

Those suffering with uncorrected hearing loss...

- Suffer chronic hypertension and CVD events twice as often as normal hearing individuals (Parana University, 2006)

- Utilize medical services five times as often as normal hearing individuals (VA, 1999, 2005)

- Up to 92% of those diagnosed with Alzheimer's suffer uncorrected hearing loss (Chartrand, 2004; University of Pittsburgh, 1999)

Discussion: Alzheimer's Disease should be rare in the elderly population today. Yet because of societal trends, including increasing rates of untreated hearing loss, pervasive loss of nutrition in the food supply, polypharmacy, and erroneous diagnostic and treatment models, Alzheimer's is *reportedly* exploding in the older adult population. As vested interests relative to each of these negative trends gain a stronger financial foothold, backed by endless yet fallacious research, seniors and their physicians find themselves almost swept up in the race to increase "market" for Alzheimer's Disease. **Caution:** The material of this chapter is meant only as consumer education, and does not constitute diagnosis or treatment in individual cases. *Before medications are changed or discontinued, it is advisable to consult with one's physician.*

Wrong Diagnostic Model

Because Alzheimer's is diagnosed with a series of tests given verbally at 3-5' @65 dB, the disregard of one's hearing acuity makes almost any diagnoses inconclusive. If you are diagnosed with Alzheimer's and were not required first to have your hearing tested and resulting hearing loss corrected *before* the tests are administered, it is more than likely that your primary problem is hearing loss, not Alzheimer's. Hearing loss causes not only communication challenges but also memory and cognitive challenges. Other contributing factors will also be reviewed here. In all cases, all such contributors *should* be explored and eliminated *before* a true clinical diagnosis can be rendered. Anything less constitutes professional negligence, ignorance, or malfeasance. Never, ever accept such diagnosis until the auditory component is measured and corrected, and cognitive factors are re-evaluated.

Wrong Treatment Model

Current theory states that amyloid plaques and tangles of tau in the brain are the *primary cause* of Alzheimer's, yet an emerging body of research suggests that these neurological aberrations are at best *secondarily involved* as immunological responses from more serious underlying causes (such as dehydration, adrenal depletion, heavy metal accumulations, medication side/interaction effects, organic nutritional deficiencies, substance abuse, and acidosis).

Alzheimer's Medications Can be Bad for Your Health!

The reduction or slowing of the formation of amyloid plaques and tau will *not, in and of itself,* improve memory. But, it can cause even more and faster cognitive and health decline. Prescribed AD medications have *not* demonstrated substantive improvements in memory, and claims slowing memory loss are not demonstrated in long-term studies.

However, these medications can seriously weaken immunology, and in many cases, speed progression of dementia. In spite of early indications that these medications can be dangerous in the long-term, their clinical human trials were "fast-tracked" in mere 6-8 weeks without knowing what they will do or for test subjects over the long haul. When overlaid with other medications, the effects can be particularly serious. The most commonly prescribed AD medications today are cholinesterase inhibitors (i.e., Aricept, Exelon, Reminyl, etc.), which exhibit the following side-effects:

•Negative changes in vision or balance,
•Dark yellow or brown urine
•Dizziness, fainting spells, uncontrollable movements, falls
•Increased frequency in passing urine or incontinence
•Muscle pains, nervousness, agitation
•Pain in the stomach or abdomen, vomiting, diarrhea
•Sweating, skin rash or hives, yellowing of eyes or skin
•Slowed heartbeat or palpitations (causing pace-maker?)
•Dry mouth, indigestion, loss of appetite, and nausea
•*Confusion, memory loss*

Urgency to Report Medication Side-Effects

If you or a loved one experience any of the above or other side/interaction/withdrawal effects it is imperative to report same immediately to your health professional. Essentially, just about all medications produce side effects, and have additive or negative interaction with each other (interaction effects).

These effects become stronger over extended periods of time. This is because medications are actually toxic to the body as the liver processes them, and the body gives up amino acids (borrowed hormones dopamine, serotonin, and melatonin) to produce the predicted effects of the medications. To use these medications the body requires a normally functioning liver and kidneys, and a plentiful supply of the hormones from which amino acids can be borrowed—these qualities are in short supply in much of the older population! Over extended periods of time, medications generally lose their beneficial effects, and then side effects increase, especially in older adults who already have reduced liver capacity, and declining immunology. Very few medications have ever been tested on the old or the young populations, but nearly always are tested on non-smoking, uncomplicated cohorts in the 22-42 age range.

Hence, slight side-effects today can become serious side-effects over time. Many of today's pathologies (Parkinson's, fibromyalgia, peripheral neuropathy, diabetes mellitus, multiple sclerosis, ALS, lupus, etc.) are virtually exploding today because of over-prescribing of medications (polypharmacy), and a virtual blackout in truly searching for and amelioration of underlying causes.

Therefore, it is incumbent for consumers to carefully study the side/interaction/withdrawal effects of every medication they are prescribed before taking them. Then, when effects do happen they will know to report them to their physician.

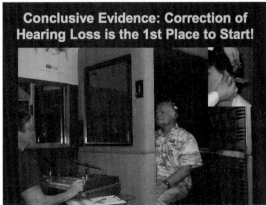

Conclusive Evidence: Correction of Hearing Loss is the 1st Place to Start!

Caution: Most medications are especially and always more dangerous for those who smoke, use high levels of caffeine, alcohol, contraindicated medi-

cations, heavy metal accumulations, and/or illicit drugs, such as marijuana, opiates, and methamphetamines. Those suffering from heavy metal accumulations and/or micronutritional deficiencies can also expect adverse reactions or contraindications to most prescription medication.

Overview of Effective Treatment Modalities

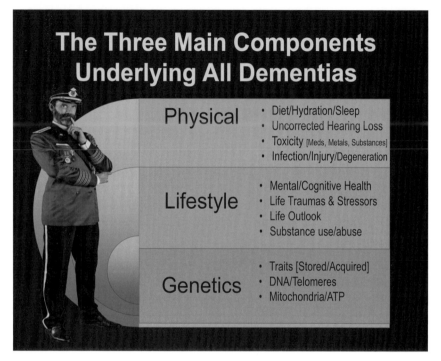

The Three Main Components Underlying All Dementias

Physical	• Diet/Hydration/Sleep • Uncorrected Hearing Loss • Toxicity [Meds, Metals, Substances] • Infection/Injury/Degeneration
Lifestyle	• Mental/Cognitive Health • Life Traumas & Stressors • Life Outlook • Substance use/abuse
Genetics	• Traits [Stored/Acquired] • DNA/Telomeres • Mitochondria/ATP

Below, are five recommended treatment pathways found to slow or reverse dementia in older adults. Each of these are described in greater detail in other resources relative to this seminar:

1. First and foremost, it is essential that every older adult where Alzheimer's Disease (AD) is suspected have their hearing thoroughly tested and any indicated hearing loss corrected immediately. In this author's firm opinion, it is nothing short of professional malfeasance and neglect for anyone to render a diagnosis of AD without ascertaining this first step is taken. In fact, auditory rehabilitation needs to be rendered as a matter of course for all older adults who have AD. For it is virtually impossible to separate a central auditory or auditory deprivation component, such as phonemic regression, without rehabilitation.

2. Next, a heavy metal assay or biomarker assessment can reveal if there are possible accumulated heavy metals. Today, high levels of deeply stored lead , mercury, cadmium, radium, arsenic, cyanide, and formaldehyde are rampant in the population at all ages (from the air, water, food, dental work, occupational hazards, and contact exposure). Heavy metals cause learning disabilities and developmental delays in children, yet are routinely ignored; and produce dementias, rheumatoid arthritis, liver damage, diabetes, CVD, and neuropathies in older adults, and again are ignored by most practitioners. Blood tests rarely show lead or cadmium that is stored in the bones, so one cannot rely on blood tests to determine the presence of some metals. When evidenced, instead of medicating for their effects, they should be chelating these from the body as quickly as possible.

3. Dehydration is rampant in society today, and particularly affects older and younger individuals. Besides too little water intake, chief culprits are medications that dry us out, lack of Omega 3 & 9 in diet, infections, and systemic/ metabolic failure. Other nutritional deficiencies, underlying pathologies, and allergies (particularly gluten intolerance) have also been implicated. Caffeine is a diuretic, and is a major cause of chronic dehydration. If brain scans indicate a shrunken brain, elimination of caffeine, reductions in meds, canola oil, gluten products, and changes in diet, including no microwaving, are a must.

4. A complete nutritional and dietary regime needs to be carefully explored for every individual suspected of AD or dementia. This would also involve removal of offending food additives, such as monosodium glutamate (MSG), Aspartame, preservatives, and minimizing synthetic vitamins and inert minerals. Such nutrition supplements as Niacin, L-Arginine, MCHC, EPA-DHA, QGel, CM Plus, Methyl B-12, Aller-B, and micronutrients are advised for nearly all older adults suspected of AD. Coupled with nutrition is an effective exercise program, and a focus on restorative sleep.

5. Addressing Underlying Disease. Since few of today's medications have actually been tested and designed for long-term use, it should be the goal of every older adult to work with their physician in eliminating the long-term use of most medications (there are exceptions). Studies show a strong correlation between good health and longevity and the number of medications taken. Hence, robust, healthy older adults take no medications, while the sickest suffer from polypharmacy! Medications, as a rule, do not heal *chronic disease*, but are instead designed for *acute disease*. Infections of the teeth (periodontal, abscesses), ears (keratosis obturans, OME) and spine (stenosis, bone spurs, scoliosis) are quite common and can be overcome. Otherwise, these become life-threatening over time. Septic keratosis obturans, for instance, is most often mistaken by medical professionals as impacted earwax, when instead, have the very real potential for becoming as deadly as a diverticulosis or appendicitis.

Note: Monographs by Dr. Chartrand cover hundreds of topics explaining how one may benefit from adult stem cell healing with cutting edge treatment approaches. For more information, contact: DigiCare Behavioral Research, 820 W. Cottonwood Lane, Suite #6, Casa Grande, AZ 85122, (520)509-6380.

For more info: **www.drmaxchartrand.org**

XVII

How to Stop or Soften
Ringing of the Ears!
(Tinnitus: "Pain in the Ear" not to be ignored)

Just a few short decades ago, tinnitus—described as ringing, buzzing, roaring, crickets, and other noises in one's head—was medically considered an *auditory hallucination,* or a subcomponent of a psychiatric disorder. Now, zoom forward to the fantastic 2010s and what do we find? Not much change. The routine prognosis for those suffering life-interrupting 24/7 tinnitus are told that "there's nothing that can be done about it", and "you just have to learn to live it". Not very enlightened considering that today few human maladies have been researched and dissected as much as this still relatively understood condition.

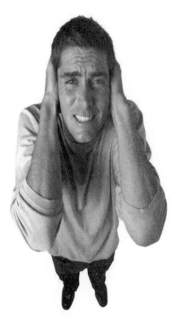

The problem is that tinnitus is not a disease or even an illness in its own right. Nor is it just one thing. It is several underlying issues coalescing at once. It is a symptom, albeit an aggravating one. It is caused principally by advancing hearing loss, starting usually in the high frequencies and progressing

Contributors of Long-Term Tinnitus
re Multimodal Tinnitus Management Model

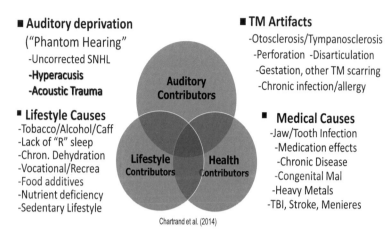

■ **Auditory deprivation**
("Phantom Hearing"
-Uncorrected SNHL
-Hyperacusis
-Acoustic Trauma

■ **Lifestyle Causes**
-Tobacco/Alcohol/Caff
-Lack of "R" sleep
-Chron. Dehydration
-Vocational/Recrea
-Food additives
-Nutrient deficiency
-Sedentary Lifestyle

■ **TM Artifacts**
-Otosclerosis/Tympanosclerosis
-Perforation -Disarticulation
-Gestation, other TM scarring
-Chronic infection/allergy

■ **Medical Causes**
-Jaw/Tooth Infection
-Medication effects
-Chronic Disease
-Congenital Mal
-Heavy Metals
-TBI, Stroke, Menieres

Auditory Contributors

Lifestyle Contributors

Health Contributors

Chartrand et al. (2014)

backwards into the low frequencies with the passage of time and continued declining hearing acuity. In about 65-70% of cases it usually starts as a high pitch tone at around 4KHz or a multiple of it (6KHz, 8KHz, 12KHz). If one corrects the hearing loss with a wide band hearing device that stimulates the cochlea beyond the center band frequency of the tinnitus, most of the problem is resolved.

Leaving out correction of the hearing loss and other health/ lifestyle factors driving it (auditory deprivation, loud noise, chronic dehydration, infection and inflammation, medication side and main effects, and diabetes type 2 and its treatment, to name but a handful) the tinnitus becomes more intense, the bandwidth of aggravating sound widens as the hearing loss moves downward in frequency, and tends to recruit more hair cells to make matters worse yet. An irony here is that if the hearing loss is left uncorrected, hyperacusis (oversensitivity to sounds) often develops, adding an additional aggravating factor. The oversensitivity usually resolves *after* appropriate hearing aid amplification is utilized. While 3-peak (wide-band) devices help, standard, single-peak devices provide marginal relief, if any.

Prevalence & Aggravation. For an idea of how aggravating and relevant tinnitus has become in today's society: According the American Tinnitus Association (ATA), at least 50 million Americans suffer from it, with 12 million suffering enough to lower quality of life and even driving some to suicide. A recent tinnitus sleep-study suggests that the effect of relentless tinnitus on the amount of glucose burned in the brain during sleep is akin that used while reading a book all night long! A mind that would prefer to drift and rest is instead processing at a clip.

Looking at it through different pathological perspectives, chronic health conditions known to contribute *to* tinnitus aggravation and to which tinnitus is known to contribute in the literature involve the Mind-Body/Body-Mind conditions of:

Mind/Body Relationships
Cardiovascular inflammation/Immunological Compromise
Hypertension/Palpitations/Arrhythmias
Transient Ischemic Attacks (TIAs)
Chronic Adrenal Fatigue Syndrome
Abnormal weight gain/weight loss
Insomnia/Sleeplessness/Sleep Apnea
Allergy/Hypoxia/COPD/Asthma
Cortical Inflammation/Idiopathic Tremors
Dyspepsia/Acid Reflux/Colitis
Hearing Impairment/Hyperacusis/Recruitment
Vertigo/Vestibular Dysfunction/Meniere's
Blurred Vision/Visual Problems
Headaches (migraines etc.)

Body/Mind Relationships
Inability to focus/Attentional Deficit Disorder (ADD)
Social/Occupational/Educational loss
Clinical Depression/Suicide Ideation/Suicide
Anxiety/Panic Disorders
Exaggerated Startle Reflex
Explosive Anger/Emotional Disorders
Memory disorders

Paranoia/associative disorders
Lethargy/Brain Fog
Obsessive Compulsive Disorder (OCD)
Personality Disorders
Factitious Disorders (Hypochondria, etc.)
Accident Prone Behaviors

Viewed through "the chicken and egg" conundrum, the lists go on and on, negatively impacting quality of life and happiness that would be difficult for those not suffering from relentless tinnitus to understand. But the toll is are *real*, the physical reactions as strong as the mental ones. ***Now, let's look at the cascade of physiological and psychological behaviors that can occur over time:***

- Progressive high frequency sensorineural hearing loss causes a high pitch tinnitus at 4KHz
- Tinnitus grows louder as hearing loss worsens, reducing cellular oxygen & bringing sleep apnea
- Sleep apnea brings sleeplessness and lethargy, bringing inflammation & attentional difficulties
- Hypoxia brings depression, anxiety, and, over time, mild pseudo pericarditis around the heart
- This progresses over time, raising blood pressure, and bringing edema to lower extremities
- Ultimately disruption of quality of life result from uncorrected hearing impairment & tinnitus

Now, let's reverse the process that occurs when we correct the tinnitus aggravation. Note the cascade back to a state of homeostasis:

- Correction of hearing loss (re F2 >10K-12KHz) *inhibits* tinnitus annoyance by about 80%
- Other lifestyle/nutritional/medical issues resolve concurrent with optimized hearing acuity
- Cardiovascular tension reduces, lowering blood pressure

CHARTS FOR EASY ANALYSIS OF YOUR TINNITUS

From the left-hand column of the chart below, what closest describes your tinnitus?

Verbal Description	Frequency Band	Mechanism	Explanatory Notes
Steady Ringing	Discrete center band @3KHz-4KHz	Functional	Active cochlear hair cell destruction re progressing sensorineural loss
Ring+pulsation (crickets)	Discrete 2KHz with broadband pulse	Functional & Structural	Microvascular (@TM and/or stria vascularis) w/ sensorineural loss
"Locusts" (Big Crickets)	Discrete 1K-1.5K Hz with broadband pulse	Functional & Structural	Same as above but progressing into lower frequencies
Wavering pitch	Discrete 800Hz-1.2KHz (unstable)	Functional	Same manifestation but loss progressing into mid frequencies
Frying, hissing noise	Broader band 500-1.2Hz (stable)	Functional & Structural	Severe microvascular constrictions with (auditory) hair cell damage
Buzz	Broader band 150-500Hz (DL expand)	Functional/ structural	Progression into lower Hz OR microvascular at stria vascularis
Roar	Broadband 60-180 Hz	Structural	Meniere's in cases of HL OR IE Viral Infection in cases of NH
All of the Above	All of the Above	Structural & Functional	All of the above plus!

From the left-hand column (below), what best describes when you hear your tinnitus?

Verbal Description	dB >Threshold	Explanatory Notes
"Just when I lay my head on my pillow"	1-3dB	Very mild, constant, usually associated with HL >4KHz
"In quiet only"	3-5dB	Mild, constant, usually associated with HL >3KHz
"Most of the time except in noise"	5-8dB	Moderate, constant, but fluctuates re HL >2KHz
"All of the time, distracting"	8-12dB	Moderately severe, constant, larger fluctuations re HL >1KHz
"Very loud, keeps me awake!"	12-15dB+	Severe, constant, very large fluctuations re HL >500Hz

- Depression/anxiety lifts, attentional deficit resolves, cellular oxygen returns @99-100% @55-65 bpm
- Back pain, headaches, sleep apnea, psychosocial issues ease over time as normal quality of life is restored

The author has been on the forefront of applied research in tinnitus for more than 40 years. He was one of the earliest professional members when the American Tinnitus Association (ATA) was formed in the late 1970s, and has served for years on its Advisory Committee as well as that of the Better Hearing Institute and the state licensing board for audiologists, speech pathologists, and hearing aid dispensers. His work has led to major inroads into understanding the relationships between tinnitus & chronic health conditions.

He has long maintained that appropriately fitted amplification, recognizing loudness growth and distortion idiosyncrasies, which define every sufferer of tinnitus and hearing loss, is the place to start in cases where hearing loss also exists, *especially in cases of high-frequency loss.*

Any other approach psychotropic, neuroleptic, CNS depressant medications not only prolong the problem but add new health challenges in the long-term. It can be a challenge to resolve threshold losses that are caused by amino-glycoside antibiotics and other toxic medications, amplification correction can still provide significant improvement in the resulting tinnitus and hyperacusis cases.

In recent years, uncountable sufferers have enjoyed significant relief from the aggravation of tinnitus and hyperacusis by using the author's approach that is trademarked **Multimodal Tinnitus Management** (MTM). MTM involves addressing the three contributive factors: 1) wide-band devices to correct the hearing loss, 2) improvements in lifestyle, nutrition, sleep, and hydration, and 3) receiving appropriate medical/health attention, as indicated.

Note: Monographs by Dr. Chartrand cover hundreds of topics explaining how one may benefit from adult stem cell

healing with cutting edge treatment approaches. For more information, contact: DigiCare Behavioral Research, 820 W. Cottonwood Lane, Suite #6, Casa Grande, AZ 85122, (520)509-6380.

When it comes to resolving tinnitus, it is a futile effort trying to find a single remedy that does not first consider and address these three contributing factors. The author's advice is to start with a hearing test and a trial on wide-band (open) amplification. Then, you can address each issue as they present from there.

XVIII
Caffeine Intoxication & Withdrawal:
Growing Public Health Menace

Introduction: *Products containing caffeine, arguably the world's most psychoactive drug, are surpassed only by sales of petroleum products worldwide. Caffeine consumption has increased among all age groups, even down to toddlers innocently sipping on 16 oz. Big Gulp Colas, so much so that growing*

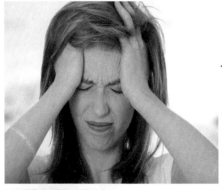

attention is turning to both the short-term and long-term serious health effects of high caffeine consumption. This chapter explores the negative psychological and physiological impact caffeine can have on various subsets of the population, and the need for greater consumer and professional education to better recognize

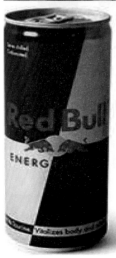

these effects. In particular, alarm over the growing incidence of caffeine Intoxication and caffeine withdrawal, including caffeine-induced anxiety, are fast making their way into recognized clinical diagnosis and treatment protocols, including the DSM-IV-TR (APA, 2000, 2012). Diagnoses for these conditions may be made based upon case history and observation of possible secondary conditions. Treatment involves avoidance and/or reduction of caffeine, counseling, and an holistic approach to improved health.

Defining Caffeine Intoxication

Etiology of caffeine intoxication (CI) arises from pharmacological stimulation of the human central nervous system (CNS), heart rate, voluntary muscle control, and other physical processes, such as diuresis and gastric secretions (Lande, 2005). Increased systolic blood pressure and analgesic effects are also noted in physical effects of caffeine ingestion (Keogh and Chaloner, 2002). Psychological and physical effects include an array of effects, from which indications of five or more may constitute a diagnosis of CI during or after caffeine use (DSM-IV-TR, 2000):

- ✦ **Nervousness, Muscle Twitching**
- ✦ **Restlessness, Insomnia**
- ✦ **Tension/Migraine Headache**
- ✦ **Adrenal Fatigue**
- ✦ **Diuresis, chronic edema**
- ✦ **Gastrointestinal disturbance, IBS**
- ✦ **Rambling thought or speech**
- ✦ **Tachycardia or cardiac arrhythmia**
- ✦ **Periods of inexhaustibility**
- ✦ **Psychomotor agitation**
- ✦ **Attention deficit behaviors**

Differentiating criteria involve whether the above symptoms are serious enough to cause "clinically significant distress or impairment in social, occupational, and other important areas of functioning" (Lande, 2005, p. 3). Most effects are expressed in terms of behavioral patterns, but anxiety is likely the most common manifestation, followed by withdrawal symptoms of mild depression, headache, irritability, difficulty concentrating, and flu-like symptoms. Hence, caffeine withdrawal (CW) tends to be the after-effects to CI, lasting up to 2-3 days or longer following

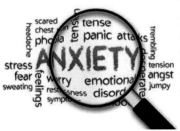

cessation of caffeine ingestion (Haskell et al., 2005; WebMD, 2004).

The degree of severity appears to be based upon four main factors: 1) body weight, 2) dose consumed, 3) individual tolerance or vulnerability to adrenal fatigue, and 4) any pre-existing psychiatric and/or medical conditions and medications (Whitsett, 1984). Peak plasma levels present about one hour after ingestion, with a half-life of 4-6 hours, depending upon body weight. Caffeine absorbs readily into body fluids and tissues, and may stimulate the body's central nervous system over a period of up to 12 hours.

Deleterious effects are noted in high doses of caffeine during interaction with many prescription medications, especially diuretics, antiasthmatics, and antidepressants. Lingering effects at the end of this cycle can cause irritability and insomnia in some individuals for days afterwards. Trait personality disorder subsets tend to show the most dramatic psychological and emotional responses to psychostimulation, and therefore must be diagnosed within an individual context. For that reason, evidence suggests frequent mis- or over-diagnosis for some psychiatric non- or pre-existing psychological conditions, such obsessive-compulsive disorder (OCD), schizophrenia, panic or anxiety disorder, attentional deficit with hyperactivity (ADHD), hypochondria, somatic delusions, post-menstrual syndrome, anorexia, etc. In other words, CI may exacerbate or present a false positive in some individuals with these conditions (Bailey, 2006; Whalen, 2005; Chartrand, 2004). Other studies link CI and CW with cases of mild clinical depression (Werbach, 1999).

Promoting increased public health threats, such as increased caffeine toxicity and GMO high fructose corn syrup, worldwide commercial interests appear to be working toward increasing market size and reach of those most vulnerable to caffeine addiction: ***The very young—and too many parents seem not recognizing this terrible threat to the health of their children!***

One of the most brazen attempts to grow a larger market of consumers is the widespread practice of negotiating lucrative two-way contracts between U.S. public school districts and commercial bottling companies, such as Coca Cola, PepsiCo, etc. to provide soft drink vending machines throughout the hallways of the schools everywhere, especially sales of high-caffeine popular drinks. Many of these popular drinks rival the notorious Red Bull drinks with four, five, even six times the caffeine contained in Coca Cola. Consequently, caffeinated drink sales to school age children have exploded to record highs and have raised considerable concerns among health agencies and professionals.

While rising obesity and pre-diabetic tendency in youth garner much concern today, there are also those concerned over deleterious behavioral effects as a result of exploding caffeine dependency, which can—coupled with increasing sugar intake --translate into serious behavioral and academic challenges (Abigail Trafford, 1999). Couple the trend with almost a universal transition toward GMO high fructose corn syrup sweetener in perhaps 80% of prepared food and soft drink products today, and it is no wonder chronic disease is exploding in the general population today (Gucciardia, 2012; Princeton University, 2010)

American University conducted a study in which its investigators concluded that the results "shows very nicely that the effects of caffeine withdrawal are consistent, that several symptoms are of large magnitude, and that a minority of people cannot perform daily functions when they go without caffeine [after reaching addicted state]" (WebMD, 2004, p. 1). Whereas 100 milligrams is enough to evoke marked withdrawal symptoms, the average person in the U.S. today consumes 280 milligrams daily, or the equivalent of two-three cups of coffee or 3-5 soft drinks. Increased worldwide sales of coffee, chocolate, and over-the-counter headache and dietary products containing large amounts of caffeine attest to saturation into nearly all age groups and walks of life (Dawidowski, 2002).

Interactions with other drugs is also of grave concern, especially in non-medical uses, such as over-the-counter weight loss products with phenylpropanolamine, and smoking cessation products containing the active ingredient of nicotine (Choice Changes, 2003; Swanson, 1993). Cases of asthma and bipolar symptoms have reportedly been aggravated or triggered by caffeine intake (Anonymous, 2006; Answers.com, 2006; Whetsell and Shapira, 1993). Sleep can be interrupted by consumption of about 200 mg. in most people, while toxic effects are prevalent in susceptible individuals at 1 gram or more per day. Prolonged use of caffeine, especially in exclusion of adequate nutrition, and/or abrupt cessation, can trigger serious toxic reactions in such individuals (Lande, 2005; Baker, 2000; Lamberg, 1999).

Testing for caffeine toxicity mostly involves case history and by eliminating other causes, such as concomitant drug-use. Blood tests for caffeine are generally not practical or even helpful in diagnosis. Thyroid studies for developing hypothyroidism may shed further light. Otherwise, symptoms such as insomnia, cardiac irregularities, and other symptoms described above may be factored into a diagnosis of either caffeine intoxication or caffeine withdrawal, depending upon which side of use history and symptomology diagnosis is rendered. Diagnoses for psychiatric conditions relative to those described in DSM-IV-TR (2000) can help identify trait personality and other mental disorders.

While *Mosby's Manual of Diagnostic and Laboratory Tests* (Pagana and Pagana, 2002) does not list any specific tests for CI or CW, there are several tests that may reveal secondary chronic disease effects that can arise from long-term caffeine intoxication, such as:

☐ Chronic mild to moderate dehydration via measurement of Antidiuretic hormone ADH tests, compared to plasma sodium levels.

☐ Immunosuppression and/or adrenal insufficiency or depletion via C-reactive and Adrenocorticotropic hormone stimulation (ACTH Stimulation) tests

☐ Caffeine-triggered allergy or asthmatic response via tests for IgE, IgG, etc.

☐ Tests for inflammation via cytokines IL-4, IL-5, and IL-6

Treatment may consist of avoidance and/or significant reduction in caffeine ingestion, and by addressing any of the above (secondary) conditions. One must keep an eye toward gradual health improvements, and hence, improvements in the secondary conditions, as well, that may require adjustments or gradual decreases in medications. Counseling and/or psychotherapy relative to functional and psychological issues will also be needed in cases of trait personality disorders. But, looking at the larger picture of public health concerns, consumer education, as well as advancement in diagnostic and treatment regimens, may actually serve to be the best remediation for all concerned.

Note: Monographs by Dr. Chartrand cover hundreds of topics explaining how one may benefit from adult stem cell healing with cutting edge treatment approaches. For more information, contact: DigiCare Behavioral Research, 820 W. Cottonwood Lane, Suite #6, Casa Grande, AZ 85122, (520)509-6380.

References

Abigail Trafford, (1999, March 23). Health Talk with Abigail Trafford. The Washington Post.

APA,(2000). Diagnostic and Statistical Manual of Mental Disorders, Fourth Edition, Text Revision (DSM-IV-TR). American Psychiatric Association, Arlington, VA: American Psychiatric Publishing, Inc., ISBN 0-89042-024-6.

Anonymous, (2006). Eicosanoids and asthma. Retrieved on April 28, 2006, from http://glorioushealth.tripod.com/asthma.htm.

Answers.com, (2006). Bipolar disorder. Retrieved on April 28, 2006, from http://www.answers.com/topic/bipolar-disorder.

Bailey, E., (2006). Is it really ADD? 10 Medical Conditions that Share Similar Symptoms as ADD/ADHD. Your Guide to Attentional Deficit Disorder. About, Inc.

Baker, M., (2000, August 2). Hazards Identification. Retrieved on April 28, 2006, from http://www.chem.tamu.edu/class/ majors/msdsfiles/msdscaffiene,htm.

Chartrand, M.S. (2004). ADHD & Kids: What's Going On? Audiology Online, retrieved on May 2, 2006, from http://www.healthyhearing.com/library/article_content.asp?article_id=217.

Choice Changes, (2003, March 9). Phenylpropanolamine Re-

call. Retrieved on April 28, 2006, from http://
www.choicechanges.com/print.php?sid=231+231&
MDPROSID=06822bOe7ece75d78bfd.

Dawidowski, K., (2002, April). Caffeine Overload. American
Demographics, Ithaca, 24(4): 16.

Gucciardia, A. (2012). Report on the UCLA High Fructose
Corn Syrup Memory Study. http://naturalsociety.
com/high-fructose-corn-syrup-damages-learning-abilities-
memory/

Gucciardia, A. (2012). Report on the UC-Davis High Fructose
Corn Syrup Study. http://www.naturalnews.com/
study.html.

Haskell, C.F., Kennedy, D.O., Wesnes, K.A., Scholey, A.B.
(2005). Cognitive and mood improvements of caffeine consumers and non-habitual consumers of caffeine. Psycho-
pharmacology, in press.

Keogh, E., and Chaloner, N., (2002, December). The moderat-
ing effect of anxiety sensitivity on caffeine-induced hypoal-
gesia in healthy women. Psychopharmocology, 164(4): 429
-431.

Lamberg, L., (1999, March 10). Brew It or Chew It? Military
Seeks Ways to Caffeinate. Journal of the American Medical
Association, 281: 885-886.

Lande, G., (2005, July 7). Caffeine-Related Psychiatric Disorders. Emedicine. Retrieved on May 2, 2006, from http://
www.emedicine.com/med/topic3115.htm.

Pagana, K.D., and Pagana, T.J., (2002). Mosby's Manual of
Diagnostic and Laboratory Tests, Second Edition. St.
Louis, MO: Mosby, Inc., ISBN 0-323-01609-X.

Princeton University (2010). A Sweet Problem: Princeton researchers find that high-fructose corn syrup prompts considerably more weight gain. http://www.princeton.edu/
main/newsarchive/S26/91/22K07/.

Swanson, J.A., (1993). Caffeine and nicotine: A review of their
combined use, interactive effects and the impact of caffeine abstinence on tobacco cessation and withdrawal. Lo-
ma Linda University, 198 pages, AAT 9333552.

WebMD, (2004, September 30). Caffeine Withdrawal is Real.
Retrieved on April 22, 2006, from http://
www.cbsnews.com/stories/2004/09/30/health/webmd/
printable646620.shtml.

Werbach, M.R., (1999). Nutritional Influences on Mental Illness, Second Edition. Tarzana, CA: Third Line Press, Inc.,

XIX

The Crucial Truth About Long-Term
OPIOID PAIN KILLERS

It is entirely arguable that one of the greatest travesties in modern medicine is in keeping millions of Americans from recovering from chronic health conditions and injuries by over-prescribing opioid analgesics in the long-term. Safe and effective *only* in the short term, these pain killers are best used during and after surgeries, acute injuries/lesions, and in end-of-life palliative care. Otherwise, these can prevent patients from ever achieving healing and homeostasis.

Depending upon one's genetics and other health factors (i.e., cellular pH, nutritional deficiencies, heavy metal accumulations, lifestyle issues, etc.), the health benefits of opioid pain killers are generally useful for about 10-14 days, after which they begin to slow healing and lose their pain killing properties. After that, either an increase of dosage is required or the patient's pain levels rise. That is why long-term use leads millions of sufferers to black market opioids, which today is reportedly as large as the legal market itself. The social price—in broken lives, livelihood, and relationships—is one of today's most hidden tragedies. In fact, opioid use causes more suicides and deaths by over-dose than any other cause today.

Long term use of opioids causes i*schemia*, which is a condition where oxygen is cut off and concentrations of carbon dioxide destroy tissues and slow the immunological process. The principal body organ that takes the brunt of this process is the liver, the gateway organ in our immunological network. When the liver goes, everything else follows. Add other types of

Important: Pro-Inflammatory cascade* from subclinical sepsis exacerbates breathing disorders

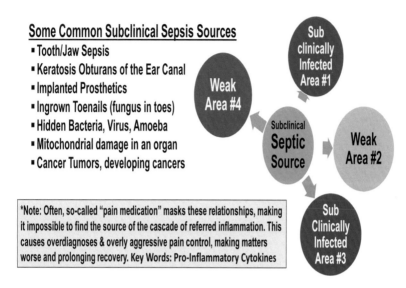

Some Common Subclinical Sepsis Sources
- Tooth/Jaw Sepsis
- Keratosis Obturans of the Ear Canal
- Implanted Prosthetics
- Ingrown Toenails (fungus in toes)
- Hidden Bacteria, Virus, Amoeba
- Mitochondrial damage in an organ
- Cancer Tumors, developing cancers

Sub clinically Infected Area #1

Weak Area #4

Subclinical Septic Source

Weak Area #2

*Note: Often, so-called "pain medication" masks these relationships, making it impossible to find the source of the cascade of referred inflammation. This causes overdiagnoses & overly aggressive pain control, making matters worse and prolonging recovery. Key Words: Pro-Inflammatory Cytokines

Sub Clinically Infected Area #3

painkillers to the opioids (see chart below) and the liver, kidneys, and developing cardiovascular disease become inevitable for ALL sufferers.

In the pain/behavioral model above, we find that as oxygen is depleted, muscle and tendon pain increases dramatically. The longer muscle and tendon pain is suffered without appropriately addressing underlying causes of illness, the more neurological issues develop, such as fibromyalgia, peripheral neuropathy, diabetic neuropathy, and, in some cases, become susceptible to lupus, multiple sclerosis, ALS (Lou Gehrig's disease), and a host of other immunocompromised neuropathic syndromes. Polypharmacy (i.e., multiple medications) *always* contributes negatively to the above milieu, so at some point, no one can be certain if the patient is really sick or just suffering a potpourri of side/interaction effects from medication overuse.

So, in *all* such cases, the real answer lies in a thorough investigation and amelioration of the underlying contributors

Diagnostic Cascade Explained

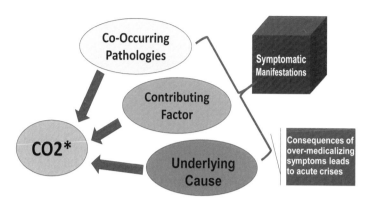

*Note: Blood Oxygen 97% & under means impending health crises.

rather than remaining on an ill-fated quest merely to "kill pain". In truth, pain is the immunological messenger that informs mitochondria that something needs attention. To "shoot the messenger" is to only delay the healing process that allows the injury/lesion to be resolved. We find the endless search for merely covering up the pain with opioids a fool's errand for the patient and nothing short of professional malfeasance or negligence on the part of health professionals.

There are only seven underlying causes to all chronic disease (see our monograph that defines these causes). Each of these should be thoroughly and honestly addressed. Lesions or injuries that cause pain, and especially infections of all kinds, should be addressed in the least invasive and damaging manner. For instance, most unrelenting chronic pain seems to be caused by unhealed injuries. Surgery is rarely the answer for most of these long-term cases, without first trying the gentle modalities of cold laser, medical massage, occupational therapy, etc. With the appropriate targeted nutrition and reduction in unnecessary medications, these modalities can bring substantial relief to almost all cases.

There are a number of available resources for those needing assistance in coming off of their opioid medicines. We have listed some resources at the end of this paper. Plus, SIRCLE staff can help.

But the larger issue is in going after and resolving underlying causes of your pain rather than attempting to circumvent them. In the following are some of the protocols that can be considered *before* going further into the murkier realm of multiple medications and invasive surgeries:

•First, address **nutritional deficiencies** by taking only live form, enterically or sublingually delivered, nutrients that have been clinically tested to resolve the deficiencies. These are

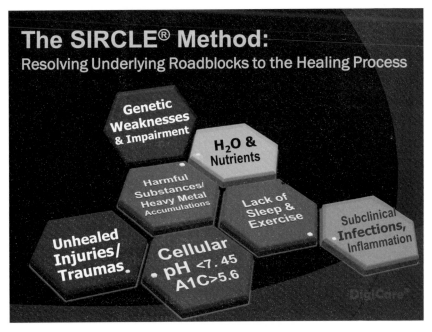

The SIRCLE® Method:
Resolving Underlying Roadblocks to the Healing Process

Genetic Weaknesses & Impairment

H₂O & Nutrients

Harmful Substances/ Heavy Metal Accumulations

Lack of Sleep & Exercise

Subclinical Infections, Inflammation

Unhealed Injuries/ Traumas.

Cellular pH <7.45 A1C>5.6

generally not available commercially. The object is to raise cellular pH from the current acidosis state of pH 6.9-7.1 to pH 7.45 where good health can happen.

•Take a **nonselective gentle, slow-acting oral chelate** over a period of three to nine months. This should be able to chelate a lifetime of accumulations of lead, mercury, aluminum, arsenic, cyanide, cadmium, and all *free form* minerals and metals from your body.

•Repair all injured areas of the body with **Deep Cold Laser** therapy and other gentle modalities that heal, not just manage your condition.

•Redistribute oxygen, and reduce necrotic fluid throughout the tissues and organs of the body and reduce intracellular/extracellular fluid and toxin accumulations with effective **Medical Message** and AromaTouch® therapies.

•**Stop microwaving food**, and instead use steaming, convection, stove top, and raw forms where possible.

•Stop use of Canola Oil and use only **Extra Virgin Olive Oil** or cold processed Coconut Oil.

•**Avoid/Minimize the following**: Gluten products (i.e., GMO wheat), High Fructose Corn Syrup (HFCS), Aspartame, Monosodium glutamate (MSG), all artificial sweeteners except for Stevia.

•**Reduce caffeine** to almost nothing (remember, you said you want to get well—-stay on the caffeine and you will not get well).

•**Get a good night's sleep** without narcotics.

•*Exercise with a prescribed regimen.* Opiate users suffer slow oxygen recovery in the muscles and have extremely overloaded livers. The best form of exercise is water-based exercise, aerobics if appropriate.

•**If you need to be admitted in a defined rehab program** at your local hospital or clinic, please do not hesitate to do so. It might be your only chance of kicking the dependency, addictions, and/or withdrawal effects.

•**Refrain from alcohol or any other narcotic or sedative** that might cause another dependency. ***Tobacco abstinence*** is a given.

•In some cases, motor function & cognition may be so impaired that **Occupational Therapy** and other therapies may be required.

...and get ready to get back your life, your health, your personal relationships, and your ability to go after your dreams!

Note: Monographs by Dr. Chartrand cover hundreds of topics explaining how one may benefit from adult stem cell healing with cutting edge treatment approaches. For more information, contact: DigiCare Behavioral Research, 820 W. Cottonwood Lane, Suite #6, Casa Grande, AZ 85122, (520)509-6380.

Website resources:

- http://www.mtv.com/news/articles/1437883/codeine-drugs-killed-dj-screw.jhtml
- http://www.vaughns-1-pagers.com/medicine/painkiller-comparison.htm
- http://wwwdasis.samhsa.gov/teds08/teds2k8natweb.pdf
- http://www.ncbi.nlm.nih.gov/pubmedhealth/PMH0001945/
- http://www.deadiversion.usdoj.gov/drugs_concern/oxycodone/summary.htm

XX

Prostate Benign Hyperplasia
The (oft) Forgotten Challenge in Men's Health

Introduction: One of Everyman's greatest fears is that he will get up many times in the night and someday find that he is... unable...to...urinate...at all. Because of a prostate grown to the size of a small grapefruit. What solution awaits him in the sparse and rude armamentarium of conventional medicine under the heading of "men's health"?

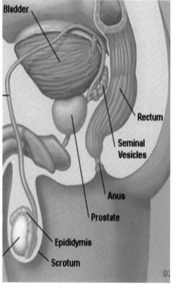

Surgical removal, and health-destroying radiation and chemo? Medications that raise risks of cancer, impotence, incontinence? Each of these "solutions" can be regarded only *slightly* better than his worst nightmare: painful and costly. Is there any hope for men doomed with...enlarged...prostates?

The Problem

The untold story of men's health is one of unbelievable risk and debilitation, incredibly high cost, poor outcomes (for the majority), and years of incontinence, impotence, and peripheral health problems they did not have before the treatments started.

Now, I grant that there are some sterling success stories out there. Many men have been successful in getting past these challenges. This is not to deny them. But for the majority, the prognoses are not so rosy. For an objective review, go

147

to http://health.nytimes.com/health/guides/disease/prostate-cancer/radiation-therapy.html. There one will find a rather benign, glossed over description of what awaits those who receive the most modern treatments, from risky radiation to painful tests and surgeries, freezing tissues, side-effect laden and cancer promoting drugs, gut-wrenching chemo therapy, and unintended collateral damage years afterwards.

The key here is to shine light on what we do BEFORE prostates get as big as buses. The next section will speak to underlying causes of prostatitis (inflamed prostrate) and hyperplasia with a brief discussion about PSA scores, so that we can look anew at their real relevance. The last section is about how we can head off the problems at the pass and stay as far away as possible from the *need* for conventional treatments.

Underlying Causes

The Top Five Causes of Death for U.S. Men: Putting it all in Perspective (CDC, 2016)

Note: The truth is that almost all men will have prostate cancer if they live long enough. After age 80 prostate cancer generally grows so slowly that many men die of the treatment of the cancer, instead of from the cancer itself. Best to first try the gentle forms of treatment, such as Crinum Latifolia, rather than starting with the invasive, risky forms of treatment.

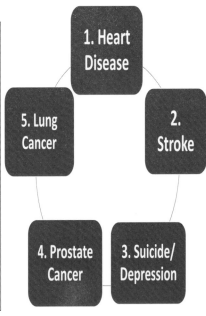

1. Heart Disease

2. Stroke

3. Suicide/Depression

4. Prostate Cancer

5. Lung Cancer

But in all cases of prostate cancer that is not yet malignant or metastasized, the place to start is to get healthy before doing anything else. Stop microwaving food, even for warming. Stop tobacco, alcohol, high caffeine, GMO wheat, high fructose, and change one's diet to one of fresh fruits and vegetables, small quantities of meat and dairy, etc.

Every man is different. Some prostates enlarge early from physical trauma to the prostate (high bicycle bars, horseback saddles, etc.). Some result from the same forces that enlarged their hearts (acidosis, inflammatory disease, chronic hypertension, medications). For yet others it is chronic disease, heavy metal accumulations, chronic dehydration, bladder and kidney disease, and/or unhealed damage to the spine. Food additives, such as Aspartame, MSG, preservatives, and synthetic nutrients are common contributors. Arguably, the worst medications for a man with acidosis and an enlarging prostate are acid reflux medications, for they cause calcium deposits in the prostate.

Just being male assures us that at some point that the prostate will enlarge. In fact, it has been said that if we live long enough virtually all men will likely develop prostate cancer at some point—albeit usually a very slow growing one that is better left untreated after a certain age. By age 40 most prostates have already grown 50% from their original walnut size. By age 50, they have usually doubled; by age 60 tripling in size is not uncommon. Between inflammation (generated from anywhere in the body) and actual cell proliferation (aka hyperplasia) over decades of living hard it is indeed a rare old-

Common Problems of Untreated or Improperly Treated Hyperplasia

- **A weak or slow urinary stream**
- **Sleep Interruption**
- **Incontinence, Urgency to urinate**
- **Bladder Infection & Stones**
- **Urethra lining damage, crimping**
- **Kidney Infections & Stones**
- **Impotence, Loss of Sex Drive**

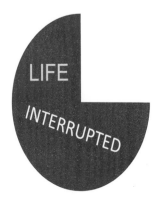

er male whose prostate is not enlarged.

For some time now, **Prostate Specific Antigen** (PSA) scores have been the clinical marker for medical attention. However, objective research studies show little correlation between the PSA score and the risk of cancer. Indeed, the tiny arsenal of conventional medications for the prostate *may* reduce PSA scores, but they also *increase* cancer risk by five-fold, in some reports. Even the $10,000+ biopsies of prostates often lead to false positives or inconclusive diagnoses. We have seen, for instance, PSA scores as high as 15.0 with no cancer, and PSA scores as low as 4.5 with full-blown cancer. Typically, we like see PSA scores of 0.0-2.0.

Here are some pointers: 1) Don't microwave your food, not even for warming, 2) avoid acid reflux by getting one's stomach acids back to pH 1.2 with Apple Cider Vinegar Caps with each meal and by avoiding gluten-rich grains, 3) strive to lower your blood pressure without medication, 4) eat an apple each day to lower cholesterol (without muscle-damaging statin drugs), 5) avoid High Fructose Corn Syrup (HFCS) where possible, 6) raise cellular iodine levels (Organic Iodine 1 drop in water daily), 7) take an organic magnesium and zinc overcome those universal deficiencies, 8) chelate with attenuated-EDTA CardioFlow to remove heavy metals from body, 9) avoid tobacco, alcohol, high caffeine, and eat fewer dairy products and smaller portions of red meat, and more fresh fruits and vegetables, and 10) floss daily & keep teeth immaculate: Doing each of these will contribute substantially toward the preventing inflammatory factors that enlarge prostates and lower your PSA score, as well as risk of prostate cancer.

To reduce/eliminate hyperplasia and inflammatory aspects (i.e., to reduce the size of one's prostate):

Take 1, 000 mg. Crinum Prostate before breakfast & before bedtime.
If you have bladder infection, take (2) U-Tract [D-Mannose]

capsules three times per day for 2 weeks; then (2) in the pm for two more weeks.

If recent history of kidney stones or kidney disease, add Cran-Caps and Ubiquinol CoQ10/PQQ per instructions of your healthcare provider.

Apply an anti-inflammatory mixture of therapeutic grade essential oils (Thyme, Cypress, Frankincense, Eucalyptus, and Clary Sage diluted with Miracell® Botanical Solution) lightly behind the scrotum (over the prostate) each night.

In addition to doing the above do the following as needed:

- Carefully read labels on food to avoid harmful substances
- Resolve all infections and fractures throughout body
- Utilize medical massage, cold laser, other modalities as indicated
- Rehydrate your body with Ionized Alkaline Water, reduce caffeine
- Follow an effective exercise regimen to improve muscle tone/oxygen
- As blood pressure etc. improves, be ready to consult with your physician on reduction of medications as indicated
- If you urinate normally during the day but have multiple trips to the restroom during the night, apply a mixture of Sweet Fennel Oil and Cypress oil lightly behind the scrotum for five or more nights in a row or until the urgency of getting up is significantly reduced to no more than once in the night.
- Never spend the night sleeping while in sitting position. Go to bed, instead.

Note: Monographs by Dr. Chartrand cover hundreds of topics explaining how one may benefit from adult stem cell healing with cutting edge treatment approaches. For more information, contact: DigiCare Behavioral Research, 820

W. Cottonwood Lane, Suite #6, Casa Grande, AZ 85122, (520)509-6380.

More Resources

Chartrand, M. (2013). *Overcoming Benign Prostate Hyperplasia* (Consumer DVD). Casa Grande, AZ: DigiCare® Behavioral Research

Princeton University (2010). A Sweet Problem: Princeton researchers find that high-fructose corn syrup prompts considerably more weight gain. http://www.princeton.edu/main/newsarchive/S26/91/22K07/.

NY Times Review (2013). Prostate Cancer Treatment Guide. http://health.nytimes. com/health/guides/disease/prostate-cancer/radiation-therapy.html.

Marcel, j. et al. (2011). Crinum Latifolium Leave Extracts Suppress Immune Activation Cascades in Peripheral Blood Mononuclear Cells & Proliferation of Prostate Tumor Cells. http://www.ncbi.nlm.nih.gov/pmc/articles/PMC3134856/

Oxford (2014). An Apple a Day Study. Retrieve from http://www.ox.ac.uk/media/news_stories/2013/131218.html.

XXI

The Modern Thyroid & the Battle Over Iodine

Introduction: Are modern homo sapiens endowed with radically bad thyroids? You would think so by the millions of Americans being diagnosed with goiter, hypothyroidism, Graves', and/or Hashimoto disease. Doubly so when one considers that learning disabilities, mental retardation, and immune diseases are skyrocketing among children, and obesity, neuropathies, and compromised immunology are exploding in the adult population—many of these as an outgrowth of the "bad modern thyroid"—or is it? The purpose of this monograph is not to diagnose or treat any individual's case, but to serve as introduction to a most complex area of a health concern that is widely misunderstood. Readers should consult with their healthcare provider before making changes to medication or treatment plan.

American's Iodine Levels are Plummeting

Approximately 70% of the body's iodine is stored in the thyroid, followed next by breast tissues, with the remainder distributed throughout every cell of the body. Without adequate levels of iodine to meet the needs of the body, serious health issues develop over time.

Studies show that Americans' iodine levels have dropped by more than 50% from levels just 30 years ago, resulting in a rise in learning disabilities and mental retardation in children, and breast cancer, obesity, fatigue, and a host of thyroid diseases among adults. Up to 90% of breast cancer is caused by the cumulative effects of x-rays!

It is not merely a matter of increasing dietary iodine, however. If it was that simple, just adding more iodine to the diet would resolve the entire problem—and there would be no need for this publication. There are also increasing levels of other substances in the food supply that compete for absorption at the body's iodine receptors.

An added issue is faulty methodology in clinical measures, T3/T4 levels in the blood, for instance, that can mask other problems, such as developing liver disease, low cellular pH (acidosis), ongoing infections, nutritional deficiencies, food sensitivities, medication side/interaction/withdrawal effects, and heavy metal toxicity. Each of these need to be considered in a comprehensive effort to address one's iodine levels.

Counting the (Correctable) Causes

But the question begs: *Why do we have so many people diagnosed with hypothyroidism these days?* Let us the count the (underlying) ways:

1) **The "Low Sodium Dietary" Trend**- Many, many cases of deficiency are a result of the campaign to dramatically reduce salt in one's diet. While high sodium in diet is not a good thing, too little can also be bad, especially in warm climate areas. Since the majority of Americans' iodine intake is from iodized salt, it is critical to add another source of iodine in one's diet proportionate to salt reduction. Using sea salt, a better source of sodium incidentally, is NOT a good replacement source of iodine.

2) **Bromine, Bromide** (in many OTC medications) and **Brominated Vegetable Oil**—used in most popular sodas and baked goods, is notorious at blocking absorption of iodine. For it occupies the same cell receptors in the body as iodine. Ten percent absorption of iodine from one's diet is the minimum absorption necessary to maintain good health and function.

3) **Chlorine or chloride**, in most public water systems, and especially in swimming pool purifying system, also comes from the halogen family of chemicals and blocks iodine absorption a the receptor level. Therefore. it is important to limit exposure to chlorine in drinking water, and in breathing it in gaseous form at public swimming pools. It is also important to avoid pools that have just been "shocked" by high levels of chlorine until such has cleared

the air and breathing is not affected by it. That can be 24-48 hours later.

4) **Fluoride**, like bromide and chloride, also blocks iodine absorption. Yet this toxin is added to public water systems with the idea that it prevents dental problems, even though objective studies show it has little or no effect in preventing dental problems. (The basis for doing this is because *naturally occurring* fluoride in minute quantities has been found beneficial). Inorganic fluoride is one of the most toxic substances known to man.

5) **Perchlorate** in the ground water has become prevalent in many areas of the country. It is industrial residue affecting ground water in at least 43 states, and is heaviest in the Lower Colorado River Basin (Yuma, AZ) where iodine levels are found to critically low in children, who suffer higher levels of thyroid issues than the rest of the nation. Even at low levels it is a known cause of mental retardation and learning disabilities, and a cause of breast cancer and neuropathic and immune disease in the general population. The studies on this are astounding, yet are unheralded in the media.

6) Finally, **"Low T3"** (also known as **Euthyroid Sick Syndrome [ESS]** and **Non-thyroidal Illness Syndrome [NTIS]**) is going virtually unnoticed in healthcare circles. This is a breakdown in the liver's ability to convert T3 due to iodine deficiency, and alkaline liver, etc. The symptoms of this syndrome range from over-diagnoses of Graves, Hashimotos, and hypothyroidism to loss of physical energy, and other life-threatening disease. Prescription thyroid medication does not address the underlying issues here.

The Answer: The SIRCLE Wellness Program

The SIRCLE Program involves at least three parties: You, SIRCLE, and your community resources. You are the one setting everything into motion and make the necessary dietary/lifestyle changes, including:

- No longer microwaving your food, not even for warming

- Carefully read labels on food to avoid harmful substances

155

- Chelation & Organic Nutrients per SIRCLE Program
- Change your swimming pool/spa water to salt water
- Avoid x-ray and CAT scans as much as possible!
- Resolution of all infections and fractures throughout body
- Utilize medical massage and cold laser as suggested
- Utilize Occupational Therapy as suggested
- Utilize Ionized Alkaline Water etc. as indicated
- Reduce commercial salt, and go with *Real Salt*, an ancient inland sea salt, which has naturally occurring nutrients in the salt with about half the sodium level.
- An effective exercise regimen that improves your condition
- As blood pressure etc. improves, be ready to consult with your physician on systematic reduction of medications as indicated

More Resources

Brownstein, D. (2009). Iodine: Why You Need It, Why You Can't Live Without It, West Bloomfield, MI: Medical Alternatives Press.

Iodine Testing Labs: FFP Lab (www.ffplab.org) 877-900-5556; Hakala Labs (www.hakalalabs.com) 303-763-6242; Labrix (www.labrix.com) 877-656-9596.

XXII
For The Children:
Extraordinary Challenges Require Extraordinary Solutions

Note: The following is excerpts from the opening chapter of the author's *How to Overcome ADHD & Other Learning Disabilities, Second Edition* (eBook format from www.amazon.com). It contains vital information that will be useful to parents and grandparents, counseling professionals, and special educators who work with developmentally delayed children. Developmental delay is an umbrella connotation that captures a wide array of conditions, *Attention Deficit Hyperactivity Disorder* (ADHD) being only a part of it. ADHD was singled out in the title because it co-occurs with many other developmental syndromes, and because it is so misunderstood by many people, even those whose business it is to know.

ADHD stands out above most other delays, because it creates socially disruptive behaviors, and because of its profoundly negative effect on the learning environment. An entire class can be disrupted, and kept from learning, for example, by the hyperactivity of just one child. Meanwhile, said child, over time, develops self-image issues and complexes that can distract from achieving their true potential later in life. Rarely does ADHD occur alone. It nearly always is accompanied with other associated conditions, such as Asperger's syndrome, developmental dyslexia, high-function autism, pervasive developmental disorder, etc. Rarely does such a child have simply one or even two aspects of underdevelopment with which to grapple, but usually must deal with physical, mental, emotional, and psychosocial challenges. Each syndrome of challenges is different; as different as the individual personalities experiencing them. For that reason it is best not to label your child with a "condition" that may mean different things to different people under different circumstances, and in fact will likely outgrow over time.

To illustrate a common scenario that seems to elude just about everyone involved in the discussion of kids and hyperactivity, let's take an example of a dilemma that uncountable parents face today: An eight year old boy we will call Brandon was referred to our clinic by a local physician. He wanted a more in-depth opinion on Brandon's case. Like many boys today who are disruptive in the classroom, the mother was told by the school that if Brandon wasn't put on the ADHD medication that he would not be allowed back into the classroom—this ultimatum, as often happens, was made before any physical or mental evaluation was conducted by anyone qualified to conduct such evaluations.

Brandon and his mother were taken to the assessment room where the little boy decided he liked my swivel chair better than the non-swivel one in which he was seated. After climbing into the preferred chair, he began twirling around and around with absolute delight, much to the consternation of an already frustrated mother.

Upon entering the room, and after hasty introductions, I grabbed the arm of the twirling chair and stopped it cold in its tracks. Then, kneeling down beside a startled wide-eyed boy, I

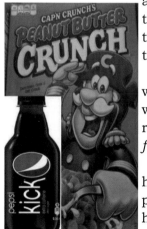

asked him what he had had for breakfast that morning. He thought for a second or two, cocked his head back and said matter-of-factly, *"Cap'n Crunch and Pepsi"*.

He was further asked if he felt that was a good, nutritious breakfast with which to start the day, to which Brandon replied enthusiastically, *"Sure! All my friends have that for breakfast."*

I then turned to the mother and asked her how she felt relative to the kind of impact that kind of breakfast would have on her son's behavior in school, to which she replied, *"Well, I hadn't thought of it that way. I guess it's not the best thing to have, but he won't have anything else."*

From there, I let the mother know—making sure the boy was hearing what was said—that such sweetened cereals are loaded with genetically modified organism (GMO) high fructose corn syrup, a highly concentrated sweetener that raises blood sugar levels to a high level and, according to at least one study, builds up fatty tissues around the heart. In addition, the high caffeine content of Pepsi Cola (combined with its own high fructose content will raise blood sugar even higher) was the equivalent of two cups of coffee and it was no wonder her little boy was so wound up.

But worse, the high from extreme sugar and caffeine sets him up for a huge crash about two hours afterwards, and "woest" be the teacher that has him in his or her class at about that particular moment. For such will surely turn hyperactivity into blatant agitation and uncontrollable behavior in one quick step! The mother was cautioned not to allow the boy to drink *any* caffeinated drinks and avoid at all costs anything with high fructose corn syrup. Instead, her son needed a high protein, raw or brown sugared or Stevia (not artificial sweetener) oatmeal or Cream of Wheat, fruit, in a quantity big enough to hold him until lunchtime. Her son also showed signs of extreme dehydration (caffeine is a diuretic, after all) and refused to drink water during the day, opting instead for *more* caffeine and sugar to create even more agitation later on.

The mother said she was not aware of any of this, and promised to make big changes to his diet, pronto. Other advice was given in addition to the above, and drugs were avoided for a much calmer, more focused boy who was allowed back into school without the mandated behavioral modifying drugs.

The above example is given to show how some simple changes in diet and parenting can make a huge difference in a child's behavior. Perhaps your child's case is not so simple. Perhaps you need to do much, much more. Perhaps the needs are greater and the behaviors more egregious. The author and his associates have long noted that many educators, administrators, and medical practitioners a lack of sensitivity and concern in getting to *causal factors.* Too often, they opt instead for the more superficial solutions that, at best, bring only temporary results. What a short-sighted world our kids live in today!

Seriously aberrant behaviors, especially oppositional be-haviors, arise largely from being labeled with something that is considered less than normal, and acted upon by what the child perceives as disrespect and being singled out in front of others. Instead of openly labeling children with conditions like *ADHD, Dyslexia, Asperger's, Autism,* etc., the adults in their lives should be focused on what *caused* the delay in develop-ment and then expend all efforts in overcoming those factors. Address them where possible and then help the child *grow past them.* But let them go their own pace; there are no defi-nite "chronological age appropriate" mileposts to achieve with-in a given time-frame. Such are man-made constructs that are useful in gauging developmental progress, but are sorely lim-ited in meaningful application when applied to a specific child.

Developmental delays do not occur in a vacuum. There are just a handful of causes, albeit an important and oft ig-nored handful that brought us to today's tragic state. Some are preventable, but *all* are rectifiable, to varying degrees. While getting to the root causes is important, more important is getting to the *solution.* Solutions abound in this book, and are found around every corner. The most effective solutions start early rather than later, but they must be started, never-theless, not postponed until all of the adults in a child's life

Introducing the Right Brain to the Left Brain

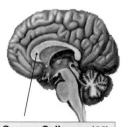

Corpus Callosum (CC) is the tiny area that connects the right & left hemispheres of the brain

1. The right hemisphere of the brain is utilized for aesthetics (art & music), emotion, expression, sees "whole".

2. The left hemisphere is used for math, deduction, abstract thought, sees only small parts of the whole.

3. CCs are smaller & less sensitive at birth in boys & take longer to develop. If the boy has chronic OME, he will likely be diagnosed with "developmental delay". With musical training & other activities all children's corpus callosums grow to full potential, raising IQ and academic performance.

are in agreement.

Likewise, this is about action, not assigning blame. It is about doing something positive, not loading them up with drugs that have tremendously negative risks and which slow, not foster true development. Children *without* developmental delays can also grow to their full potential and beyond when the same solutions are applied here, as well. So, this is not just about delayed children, but ALL children. The author is of the firm belief that today's generation can outperform any previous generation *if* the current knowledge base were put into practice. But instead, too many people are looking for shortcuts: drugs that stunt growth, well-funded programs that warehouse and coddle, labels that only garner more funding and entitlements, or serve simply as excuses as to why a child misbehaves and performs poorly. We want to pull the teeth on this kind of reasoning, once and for all, straighten up shoulders and get busy helping some kids get back onto the path to a full, rich, and exciting life.

To be clear, there are millions of earnest, hard-working youth striving to grow, learn, and be ready to take on the mantle of families and society when the time comes for them to do so. There are millions of parents who give their all for their children's successful life preparations. There are tens of thousands of skilled, dedicated special educators and therapists who strive mightily to give their charges a fighting chance to meet their fullest potential. There are classroom teachers who exert enormous amounts of energy and round-the-clock effort toward overcoming the challenges of an often desperate educational environment. There are countless administrators and staff who put their all into resolving setbacks and barriers in programs, funding, and outcomes in an often disordered and over-politicized educational system.

Not the least, taxpayers and private individuals give generously and often bequeath huge, unprecedented sums of funding toward the young with learning disorders. The caveat to this well meant generosity is that most of it is locked into the proverbial "box" of the political and social framework of our day, what we call the *Zeitgeist* of our times. This may not be all that helpful if you are one of those parents that likes to get to root causes so that your child may overcome their learning disorder without being expected to take growth-stunting, immune-stressing, and high-risk narcotic medications in the misguided effort to change behavior. For sure, these kids are not suffering from a drug deficiency. Nor are their disabilities necessarily permanent ones.

Indeed, here's something you rarely hear today: Most developmental delays are outgrown by early to mid-adulthood, the "late bloomers" they are sometimes called. How late, and how many psychosocial and self-esteem complexes develop during that period of time depends a lot on the adults in their lives. If there is a constant reminder that they are "different" they will internalize that into either a lifetime of dependency or exclusion or, worse, into passive or active rebelliousness— those without loving parental guidance sometimes go on to self-abuse with drugs, alcohol, or promiscuity. In every case where diagnosis (official or not makes little difference to them) has labeled them with a specific form of delay or disorder, they need to be reminded that theirs is just a delay in development, not rock-wall barrier. Some organizations with conflict-of-interest funding will say on their websites and literature that these are lifelong problems. We have seen too many cases that were not lifelong. Your child's case does not need to be lifelong!

If you scan history, examples of those with developmental setbacks, whether their name is Albert Einstein or Thomas Edison, or Alexander Graham Bell, Helen Keller, or George C. Scott, Mozart, Beethoven, George Bernard Shaw, et al., are replete and long. They changed history—and who would've thought? In fact, some of the greatest thinkers of all time suffered from learning and physical disabilities during their early years. But who's telling you and your child that? Instead, we hear from one of the largest associations for learning disabled children that these disorders are not curable and cannot be overcome, that these disorders will plague individuals throughout their lifetimes. I beg to differ.

This author, as a severely hearing impaired child, and later a profoundly deaf adult, has lived and worked through much of what is covered here. He sat in myriad classrooms

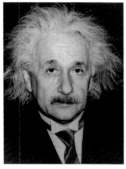

not knowing what the assignments were, nor hearing the teacher's instructions. If he sat on the front row he made A's; on the second row, B's; on the third row or further back, he often didn't know what class he was in. It was a marvel that homework was even turned in. How often his lack of hearing was judged as a behavioral issue or as a failure to pay attention! Reading two books for every one assigned was his saving grace.

Today, still deaf and aided with a multichannel cochlear implant and assistive devices, his main work is as a researcher, peer reviewer of professional journals, professor, and publisher. He spends his "spare time" leading a community jazz band to give kids and adults a chance to play great music and to achieve more and reach higher because of it. So, there you have it, those of you who suffer from developmental delay: become an avid reader, play a musical instrument, and practice daily, along with a few other special considerations, and you will grow past just about any delay or barrier thrown into your path!

Add the special advantages afforded the handicapped today as a result of the Americans with Disabilities Act (1990), and you will find an entirely new world from the one in which the author grew up. Rarely utilized properly for the deaf and hearing impaired like it should, even to this day, it enables those individuals who *do* utilize the ADA an advantage that sometimes places them out in front of even those who have no delays or handicaps.

Hence, every television program, every movie, every speech given over electronic media in the United States is closed, open, or real time captioned. In the classrooms, if requested, students can enjoy Real Time Captioning—that is far superior to signing in the classroom, where so much detail is left out. Likewise, jury duty, church and civic meetings do not have to be that impossible task it once was, as Real Time Captioning makes it possible.

Assistive technologies, coping strategies, speechreading training, hearing aids, cochlear implantation...today even a

163

deaf kid can be the next Einstein or Mozart or Edison!

But what of the ADHD or Dyslexic kid? They are often one and the same, by the way—in other words, many developmentally delayed kids have hearing loss, but too often hearing screenings miss the ones that really need help. Or the Asperger's kid. Take caffeine and high fructose out of the developmentally disordered child's diet, and watch them calm down. Check for heavy metal accumulations (blood tests will not reveal stored heavy metals, incidentally). If lead, cadmium, barium, perchlorate, mercury, etc., are found in the bones, get your child chelated immediately with a gentle attenuated chelating compound like CardioFlow.

Where do prescription drugs come into the discussion? The author considers one of modern society's more problematic practices is in arbitrarily medicating behaviors of children. Most such medication is given by court order—if only the courts understood the dangers and risks they are forcing upon our troubled young people! None of these medicines have even been trialed for efficacy and safety with young populations, yet at any given time more than 16 million American schoolchildren are forced to take these side-effect laden drugs. No wonder drug use is skyrocketing in our public schools!

Do you want to dramatically increase your newborn child's chances of developing optimally and without delay? Don't allow vaccines to be given until they are at least six months old (CDC guidelines say 12-months, but hospitals today are routinely attacking undeveloped immune systems at or near the time of birth! Remember, you the parent are the boss.

Do you want your child to get a good night's sleep and to develop better socialization with your family? Enforce a given bedtime and take the television and computer out of his/her bedroom. Want their brains to develop faster? Sign them up for band, choir, dance, voice, art, crafts—if your school has turned into a cultural wasteland like most US schools today, search out private and community-based programs that still afford the young these opportunities.

Want them to enjoy better food-to-nutrition synthesis? Stop microwaving their food (see the last chapter for a treatise on this vital topic). Tall order, but good advice if you truly want

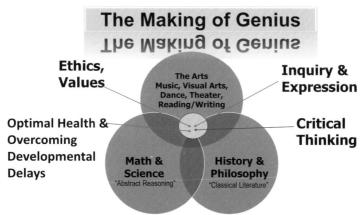

The Making of Genius

Ethics, Values

The Arts
Music, Visual Arts,
Dance, Theater,
Reading/Writing

Inquiry & Expression

Optimal Health & Overcoming Developmental Delays

Math & Science
"Abstract Reasoning"

History & Philosophy
"Classical Literature"

Critical Thinking

Elegance + Health + Holism + Coherence + Efficiency = Educational Power*

* From The Center for Arts in the Basic Curriculum, 2008

your child to stand a fighting chance in today's society. Take away the caffeinated drinks from your home refrigerator and forbid your children drink them (see the chapter on caffeine and you will experience a Eureka! Moment.

To be sure, doing the bold and daring things outlined in this book will allow your child to someday become a leader among the millions that are not enjoying the developmental benefits of the fine arts. Why are SAT scores half what they were 20 years ago, and even farther below the norm from 50 years ago? Why are today's A's about on par with C's of just 20 years ago? Why is remedial education the single largest expenditure for today's state universities? Why is functional illiteracy rampant in today's society? Why are American schoolchildren stuck at the bottom of the world in math and science surveys? Because of what has been taken out of the schools: Music, dance, art, drama, physical education in core curriculum for K-12. And it will stay that way until they are put back into the core curriculum and every child is afforded the opportunity to grow the brains that overcome developmental delays, make them reach higher than previous generations, and become all that they can be!

Your child, given the right tools and opportunities, can do the seemingly impossible. *All are children of the same divine birthright!* Indeed, every single measure of societal progress shows that our kids, and most especially our boys as a demographic, are *losing* the battle, falling further and further behind. While they are *"Waiting for Superman"*, academic expectations in too many schools are being dumbed-down, academic outcomes are declining, and our kids are getting boxed into a corner of social engineering and diminishing options to overcome their own developmental challenges! It's time to throw off the shackles, get creative, and see how far these kids can go!

For most of these challenges are due to no fault of the child, or their parents, but are simply societal trends that need changed. The goal is to awaken, to stiffen spines, and fresh courage take so that this and future generations of young people can be saved from what's been holding back the current generation. For it will take *everything* we can muster and *more* to reverse course, and to give the upcoming generation a solid platform from which true human progress can be built.

Please, remember as you read and ponder the counsel and information found here that you and your child have been through an *extraordinary* ordeal. Heartache and disappointment, tears and fears, effort that only you know has been expended. Now, it is going to take *extraordinary*, but not difficult, things to bring about a change in the right direction. Doing something *different*, even better, than the mainstream is doing; actually, doing what the mainstream *should* be doing if they want *their* children to reach their highest potential, *is* the order of the day!

Uncountable learning disabled children have been where your child is today. Every one of them found these principles to work, whether intended or accidentally. Years later, these children grew into outstanding, productive adults. They enjoyed successful families and careers. From time to time they send the author photographs of their families, and talk about their successes and achievements over the intervening decades. They have remarkable vocabularies, and are exceptionally fluent. Some own thriving businesses. Most have college degrees. Some are master teachers. They found their place in society, and brim with self-confidence and self-fulfillment. They are loving fathers and mothers, friends and neighbors. Today, they stand heads above their less challenged peers, and contribute mightily to a better world.

People who knew these children earlier are shocked and amazed. They marvel, *could it be? How did this happen?* Many school teachers and administrators, who earlier saw them as the kid who stood on chairs and made noise, shake their heads in disbelief. *This is the Johnny I knew?*

Then, they let out a sigh of relief. *This is the child I taught, umm...wow... (lump in throat)....am I ever proud to have played a part in this extraordinary person's life!*

Epilogue I to "For the Children"

The Grand Chemical Collusion: Controlling Our Children's Behavior

Some battles are so lopsided that one would be hard-pressed to find the defender when the two contenders stand side-by-side. In one corner we have the largest, most moneyed industry in the world, Big Pharma. Weighing in on the side of Big Pharma are a majority of the nation's 16,000 public school districts, the AMA, the US Department of Education, the teachers unions, and most state and federal agencies who are ostensibly charged with pro-tecting children. These are the proponents for drugging our kids to control behavior as a first line of action, before causal factors can be addressed. They are further bolstered by a cadre of coop-erating mental health professionals and many universities. Flawed studies back up their dangerous hypotheses that drug-ging the most helpless segment of our population is a preferred route in lieu of saving families, improving children's health and re-instituting the fine arts programs that help them overcome learning and developmental disorders and rise to their full poten-tial.

In the other corner, we will find millions of parents that stand alone against this Goliath of vested interests. They are bolstered by a small but growing handful of brave health professionals, medical doctors, teachers, and social workers, and independent health researchers who oppose the wholesale drugging of our children.

The vested interests, on the other hand, are the ones that when Johnny stands on his seat or talks out of turn or does poorly on his NCLB test, makes sure he is sent to a cooperating physician who will give him a once-over diagnosis based on the Connors Checklist, a prescription, and presto, Johnny becomes a financial asset to the school and is no longer a liability. The fact is, U.S. kids are the most drugged in the world—like their adult counterparts—more than all the rest of the world combined. The number would shock any objective observer: Between 13 million to 16 million kids at any given moment. The vast majority of these drugs are cocaine-class amphetamines, methamphetamines, antipsychotics, deadly neuroleptics, mind-altering anti-depressants, and powerful sedatives. Kids in incarceration are drugged at incredibly high rates, while kids in foster programs are drugged 4 to 5 times as often as kids who live with their own parents.

According to investigative reports, thousands of kids are restrained or held down while being forced to take drugs that will modify behavior, stunt development, and start them on the pathway to mental health problems that can last a lifetime. The list of such atrocities is as real as it is disgusting. This is child abuse pure and simple, and yet it often is backed by court order. The state should never be an abusive parent. There are always gentler, more effective ways for modifying behavioral without such high risks for harm.

Suicides, suicide-ideation, and homicides are many times higher in this group AFTER they have been forced into dependence on these drugs. No matter what conflict-of-interest research shows, substance abuse in this group is several times higher than in the non-drugged kids, regardless of what biased studies show on this topic. The most common type of drug forced on these kids are addictive and mind-altering ADHD stimulants that are also sold on the street, where they are injected, snorted, and abused just like their illegal counterparts. Their effects occur on the same brain receptors as cocaine. The results, over time, are the same.

Once dependent on these so-called medicines, unbelievable, excruciating violence occurs during withdrawal from these same medications. Many if not most of these kids are downing high caffeine "energy drinks" on top of a nutrient-starved diet. Every single case of extreme mass violence (Columbine, Minneapolis High, Virginia Tech I & II, Sandy Hook, Aurora, etc.) has involved these drugs in some way. Several thousand American kids have died in incidents related to these drugs, since they were brought to market. Uncountable hearts have been damaged, physical growth stunted, emergency room visits required, mental development delayed, and permanent neurological damage are found in the wake of kids being forced on these drugs, all the way down to 18 months of age. The more mentally underdeveloped (e.g., autistic spectrum) the more these dangerous drugs are administered.

Now, with the huge push by billionaire-backed initiatives at the state level all over the US to legalize marijuana, in particular, and all illegal drugs in general, drug addiction and alcoholism is at an all-time high of over 65 million in the US at this writing (2015), and that includes the "pain killer" inspired opium and heroin epidemic sweeping the nation! How a nation can long survive such rates of substance abuse is yet to be seen, but it is hoped that the parents of this nation don't wait to find out.

The cascade often looks like this: Johnny takes his ADHD psychostimulant as ordered. After he cannot sleep for days afterwards, he is given a sedative to make him sleepy. Then, we awakens mentally fatigued, partially because he failed to get Beta level of "sleep" and the narcotics are still in his system. So he starts bingeing on caffeine drinks. He's depressed, so he's finally given an SSRI/SNRI anti-depressant...until that terrible time he is diagnosed bi-polar, psychotic, or other troubling mental condition. As motor problems develop, he is then prescribed a neuroleptic or antipsychotic, and develops dyskinesia and other terrible side effects reminiscent with (young) Parkinson's. Dependency becomes a never-ending treadmill. This is the beginning of a life of polypharmacy-created pathologies. Granted, this example is among the extreme cases, but the crime is that it happens, albeit legally, and *most especially* if he is a ward of the State.

Thankfully, the vast majority of kids recognize (and fear) the way they feel while on these drugs, and usually do not comply long enough to go the entire cascade. But some, especially those in foster care or in the juvenile justice system where such drugs are routinely court-ordered, are not so fortunate. They become the most abused victims in this terrible collusion between education, government agencies, medicine, and Big Pharma. Parents, you are in charge here. Apply the principles learned in this book and don't let anyone do this to your kids. No vaccines until their immune systems are developed enough to withstand the trauma they bring (usually 6 months of age for most boys). And not too many vaccines, ever. They will build natural immunity to *most* diseases if their bodies are healthy.

Epilogue II to "For the Children"

The Power of Music:
Musical Practice & Brain Development

Children and youth who take weekly music lessons, perform with a band, orchestra, or choir, and who practice individually for at least 25 minutes or more daily:

- **Enjoy incredibly rapid brain development compared to their non-music peers!**
- **Develop higher Cognitive IQ and always rise to the top of their class!**
- **Develop Spatial IQ with advanced eye-hand coordination!**
- **Overcome learning disabilities and developmental delays!**
- **Learn socialization, organizational, and interpersonal skills that last a lifetime!**
- **Graduate and go to college in far higher numbers than non -music peers!**
- **Enjoy greater success in their life, social relationships, and chosen professions!**

More than 40% of all school children suffer from **middle ear infections** or chronic otitis media with effusion (OME) during the first three years of their lives. About 80% of these cases will be of the "silent" OME type, presenting no outward symptoms, such as fever or pain, and go undetected by the adults in their lives. Chronic OME creates **developmental delays**.

These delays may appear in the form of speech-language delay, reading difficulties (developmental dyslexia), under-development of central auditory attending and squelching skills (often mistaken for ADD), spatial skills challenges, Asperger's, and mild cognitive deficiencies that affect reading, math, and social development.

The human brain consists of two hemispheres. The **right hemisphere** is used for spatial, emotional, artistic, and holistic skills; the **left hemisphere** is used for logic, deduction, mathematics, and abstract skills. The *only* direct neurological connection between these two areas of the brain is a small band of tissue about the size of a pencil, called the **Corpus Callosum** (CC). All information between these hemispheres travel via the CC. The size and development of features of the CC during early brain development determine gender specificity and brain specialization. Its later development determines degree of intelligence. This is a lifelong process and continues to develop throughout one's life.

At birth, the CC in male newborns is about 30% smaller and less sensitive than in females. This difference appears to be help **brain specialization** in males, but places them at risk for delayed cognitive development. Girls, on the other hand, enjoy nearly equal development for both hemispheres (due to the larger dendritic mass of the CC) and are generally able to master language, communication, and fine motor skills earlier than boys (hence, the phenomena of "women's intuition"). However, boys exhibit superior visual development, faster reaction times, and greater gross total body movement skills.

However, the CC must continue to develop at a specified rate so that boys can "catch up" with girls academically, cognitively, and socially. Boys who suffer from OME during their first three years of life or more will also suffer development of the CC and other developmental areas will be two years behind their peers in reading and math, and in socialization skills. 88-92% of cases of ADHD are boys for this very reason. Contrary to current practice, prescription drugs are not the way to develop the brain. Musical training, a non-microwaved, organic diet, and plenty of sleep and exercise can help both boys and girls overcome ADHD. No caffeine or high fructose corn-syrup. Caffeine and sugar cause tremendous over-diagnosis of ADHD, incidentally.

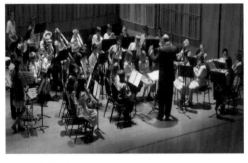

Therefore, it is absolutely crucial that music programs be put back into primary and secondary schools if America ever hopes to get back on top of the world in math, science, and reading. In fact, the long-standing decline in math and science performance of U.S. school children tracks precisely with the abolition of music programs from the years 1970 onward. Meanwhile, nations at the top of the worldwide math and science survey *ALL* feature music and the arts as core curriculum K-12. In those countries, it is not unusual to find fifth grade symphonies being led by 15-year old conductors that rival their professional counterparts. Their average students compete with our best students.

Albeit the schools that already have music as core curriculum, whether in affluent communities or the poorest neighborhoods—makes no difference—are *always* the top performing schools in their districts and states. Developing musical skills has been found to be considerably more effective than all other forms of therapy. In fact, contrary to popular thought, without musical skills development, other forms of therapy consistently show poor results. *Nothing approaches the effectiveness of taking up a musical instrument, joining a choral group, band, or orchestra, and practicing individually a minimum of 25 minutes a day.* By so doing, children will have a better chance at achieving their true potential. Furthermore, they will come closer to achieving their full potential in life.

To order ***How to Overcome ADHD & Other Learning Disabilities Without Harmful Drugs, 2nd Edition (2015),*** go to: https://www.amazon.es/Overcome-Learning-Disabilities-Without-Harmful-ebook/dp/B0145S7MC6

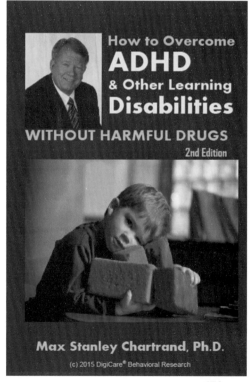

Appendix

Basic SIRCLE® Patient Checklist

Introduction: The following explains how you may optimize the outcomes of your SIRCLE® Wellness Program. They are time tested and can have a powerful influence on your success in overcoming developmental and acquired health issues. If there are questions on any of this, please feel free to inquire how it can make a difference in your ardent quest for better health for you and your family. This is not a complete list, but can serve as an adjunct to your SIRCLE® Treatment Program.

✔ **Make sure you are not wearing your cell phone anywhere near your hips as the RF radiation will weaken your hip joint and destroy surrounding tissues.**

✔ **Avoid microwaving**, even for warming food. Instead, use convection, steaming, grilling, baking, crock pot, pressure cooker, etc. for cooking methods.

✔ **Use only Extra Virgin Olive Oil** or Cold Pressed Organic Cooking Oils or Real Butter, stop using Canola and other plasticized oils.

✔ **Avoid/minimize GMO high fructose corn syrup (HFCS)**, artificial sweeteners, foods with artificial dyes and flavorings where possible. Stevia is fine. Minimize high caffeine, avoid tobacco & alcohol, other drugs.

✔ **Eat at least 50% of your daily meals with fresh vegetables, fruits, berries, nuts, and whole non-GMO grains**. *Eat an apple daily to lower cholesterol.* Reduce/minimize processed, ready processed, or packaged foods. Avoid GMO-Wheat products where possible, and most especially avoid GMO wheat bread if you are trying to lose weight. Replace regular potatoes with sweet potatoes where possible.

✔ **Drink at least 10-16 oz. filtered water every other hour** during waking hours, more if in high heat for a period of time. Ionized alkaline water will especially aid you in recovery.

✔ **Each morning--to raise transverse colon & flatten your stomach-- while in bed, do leg lifts @45°.** 5 of the left leg, 5 of the right, five of both. Then, hold legs up at 25° for 10 seconds, rest, repeat lifting up your legs several times. Other exercise: Walking (hiking), swimming (in non-chlorinated pools best), bicycle (indoor stationary bicycle), Pilates, Yoga, Cardio Kick Boxing, Zumba, etc. Don't overdo it!

✓ **Be sure to use the BMI Exercise machines faithfully.** Those who diligently do so experience MORE spinal decompression, more flexibility in their joints, better body mass index (BMI), better digestion, better sleep, and overall fitness. Those that do not will not progress as optimally.

✓ **Avoid medications (where possible) that dampen immunology** or healing, including steroids, NSAIs, opiates, nerve blocks, and others that prolong illness or can add negatively to overlay effects.

✓ **Dental health comes to the fore:** Be sure to floss daily and make sure plaques are not building up around the gums, under crowns, and around fillings. Much heart disease traces its footsteps to such considerations. *Recommend Oral-B Electric Toothbrush with On Guard Tooth Paste twice daily!*

✓ **Avoid *all* antiperspirants** (aluminum); use only mild **deodorants** (Arm & Hammer, etc.) and essential oils.

✓ **Set a strict bedtime routine** and time and follow it "no matter what" (sleep in bed rather sitting up)—avoid foams laden with allergens or positive ions.

✓ **Stay a safe distance from your electrical transformer**, high power wire, underground cable, or substation (consider getting a negative ion generator for your bedroom).

✓ **Get plenty of sunshine during the day** to reset your biological circadian cycle so that you can sleep soundly in the night. Twenty minutes of sun exposure 3x per week increases the "super vitamin D" you manufacture.

✓ **Stay a safe distance from your electrical transformer**, high power wire, underground cable, or substation (consider getting a negative ion generator for your bedroom).

✓ **Follow a therapeutically designed exercise regimen.** Remember that water exercise is best for conditions with poor oxygen/glucose recovery or neuropathic conditions.

✓ **Get plenty of sunshine during the day** to reset your biological circadian cycle so that you can sleep soundly in the night. Twenty minutes of sun exposure 3x per week increases the "super vitamin D" you manufacture.

✓ **Avoid overexposure to high chlorine**, fluoride, bromide, and other neurotoxins. Do not hesitate to adjust those items within your control or that can be requested.

Postlogue from The First Edition

For years it has amazed me when otherwise intelligent people will criticize the concepts taught here. First, my guess is that these concepts are interrupting someone's gravy train--there is certainly no danger or high-cost involved in trying what is recommended, but could mean huge losses to those who have a vested interest in an unwell population! The burden of proof is not on this author or any other author who espouses the gentle, no-risk strategies of healing. Uncountable individuals who have tried these principles and who have overcome their DMII and other chronic disease are the proof.

But, ah, they want the kind of big-dollar proof that Big Pharma must show on their potentially very dangerous drugs--the kind of drugs that rarely heal and are so laden with side/interaction/ withdrawal effects as to speed hundreds of thousands of people to early death---the kind that are so caught up in myriad million dollar lawsuits, out of court settlements, and trialed for merely 4-8 weeks, but *never* tested or designed for long-term use, the kind with effects in which immunology is suppressed and requires ever larger doses for any positive effect, or the kind that wear out the liver, the kidneys, the adrenals, the pancreas, the heart, the muscles, and deplete the bones of calcium as they plunge the body into acidosis and destruction!

No, the burden of proof is on the critics*. They* can spend the $800 million dollars on each recommended nutrient to see if it works. But, of course, they wouldn't do that.... They know that if the trials were unbiased and designed to show *long-term* results, that ailing individuals would become healthier. They know that if they required trial participants to stop microwaving, stop smoking, stop caffeine, refrain from alcohol, eat non-irradiated, non-degerminated, naturally fortified whole foods that people would get well--and stay well! People would then have the energy to start exercising, lose weight, and feel energetic again! Cancer would be rare, pervasive diabetes type 2 would become history. Babies would be born with fewer birth defects. Autism (and other developmental assaults) would become almost non-existent as it used to be, and we could begin again educating our children without Olympian-sized barriers to learning in their path like we did in the 1950s and 60s.

But, of course, they can't have that. Huge sectors of the workforce would be displaced. What would happen to the largest and fastest growing industries in the world? What would happen if all those kids soared in academic and life preparation, if people lived longer, no longer warehoused in old age with handfuls of drugs to dominate their very existence!

There is a better way. Think what would happen if a trillion or more otherwise wasted dollars per annum were infused back into the economy to make it more productive! Those workers who are displaced because people got well can go to work relieving the suffering of the seething masses of underserved throughout the world. They can improve the food and water quality, and provide true wellness counseling. They can help the tens of millions addicted to tobacco, marijuana, cocaine, narcotics of all kinds, including sleeping pills, pain killers, Ritalin, and opiates! Legitimate health follies will always exist on Mortal Earth. No way around that--but at least we can put more real research and innovation into healing and relieving suffering where it is truly needed!

Viruses will still evolve. Accidents will still happen, people will age, scheming men will plant drugs in the food and drinks to hook people on their products as they always have. Fools and the unsuspecting will buy and ingest their Trojan Horses of early death.

Type A personalities will still be prone to overwork. Type Bs will still be prone to taking it easy. So, the challenges will still be there. *For once, can those of us in the healing and helping professions be honest about it all?* Can we put vested interests aside, and design objective, *long-term* studies, and publish forthrightly on the side/ interaction/withdrawal effects of the recommended substances? Can we speak on levels of risk in a way that the consumer understands there are mild risks with misuse of natural substances--but still risks if not used intelligently--and *severe risks* with misuse of narcotics and other powerful, bullying drugs? After all, drug dealers are not breaking into health food stores. People are not dialing 911 for overdose on nutritional supplements. Can we be adults and tell them the truth?

About the Author...

Max Stanley Chartrand, Ph.D., CSP, is profoundly deaf and a cochlear implant user. He has studied, worked in, and published on topics of health for more than four decades. He has earned six advanced degrees, including two doctorates and is a professor of Behavioral

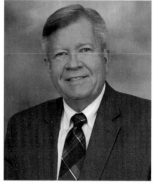

Medicine and is a writer, researcher, and keynote speaker at professional associations nationally and internationally. He has earned the highest professional credential of the National Speakers Association. In 1994, he was honored with the *Joel S. Wernick Excellence in Education Award.*

He has also served on the advisory committees to the American Tinnitus Association, the Better Hearing Institute, and Audiology Online. He is an officer on the Council for Nutritional & Environmental Medicine, an international consortium of collaborative research, and serves on the Federal & State Advocacy Committee of the International Hearing Society, and on the State Licensing Board for Audiologists, Speech Pathologists, and Hearing Instrument Dispensers.

Areas of interest in his research have been nutrition, diabetes, neuropathy, tinnitus, communicative disorders, learning disorders, cancer, and a wide range of health challenges that plague mankind.

He is deeply concerned that Americans are being made sicker by over-medicalization of symptoms at the expense of not addressing underlying causes of chronic disease. The material in this book is the result of four decades of research, clinical practice, and education in the healthcare field. The goal is to help every reader meet their full potential in leading a longer, fuller, and richer quality of life, happiness, and optimal health.

Dr. Chartrand lives in Casa Grande, Arizona with his wife Glenys Anne Chartrand, who has a background Adult Rehabilitation, Psychiatric Occupational Therapy and Age-Related Services. She is the founder of the internationally acclaimed SIRCLE® Program that was started in New Zealand almost three decades ago. Together, they developed many new and highly successful approaches to overcoming chronic disease and loss of function. They may be reached at "Contact Us" at www.drmaxchartrand.com.